Leaves as Vegetables

Food Significance and Nutritional Information

Roby Jose Ciju

CONTENTS

i

INTRODUCTION

Leafy vegetables or vegetable greens are considered to be richest source of dietary fiber, vitamins and minerals. Daily consumption of minimum 100 to 150 grams of leafy vegetables along with a main diet is recommended by many health experts for balanced nutrition of a human body. Apart from its health-providing properties many leafy vegetables are considered to have medicinal benefits also, especially those vegetable greens which are loaded with antioxidant vitamins and minerals.

An antioxidant is a substance that inhibits oxidation, especially that of free radicals. Free radicals are chemically unstable molecular fragments or atoms that are directly responsible for cell degeneration, DNA damage, malignant tumour formation (cancer) and diabetes, cataract, heart diseases and other cell degenerative diseases.

In other words, antioxidants have cell regenerating and rejuvenating properties and therefore prevent ageing process. By scavenging on free radicals, antioxidants increases body's acquired immunity against many diseases. Antioxidants are also anti-inflammatory and anti-carcinogenic.

Amaranth Leaves

Amaranth belongs to the family *Amaranthaceae*. There are several species of edible Amaranth and major among them are *Amaranthus blitum; Amaranthus cruentus; Amaranthus hybridus; Amaranthus retroflexus; Amaranthus caudatus; Amaranthus mangostanus; Amaranthus lividus* and *Amaranthus dubius*. Normally, leaves are consumed after cooking.

Nutrition in Raw Amaranth Leaves

Nutrient	Unit	Value per 100g	1.0"cup"28.0g	1.0"leaf"14.0g
Water	g	91.69	25.67	12.84
Energy	kcal	23	6	3
Protein	g	2.46	0.69	0.34
Total lipid (fat)	g	0.33	0.09	0.05
Carbohydrate, by difference	g	4.02	1.13	0.56
Calcium, Ca	mg	215	60	30
Iron, Fe	mg	2.32	0.65	0.32
Magnesium, Mg	mg	55	15	8
Phosphorus, P	mg	50	14	7
Potassium, K	mg	611	171	86
Sodium, Na	mg	20	6	3
Zinc, Zn	mg	0.9	0.25	0.13
Vitamin C, total ascorbic acid	mg	43.3	12.1	6.1
Thiamin	mg	0.027	0.008	0.004
Riboflavin	mg	0.158	0.044	0.022
Niacin	mg	0.658	0.184	0.092
Vitamin B-6	mg	0.192	0.054	0.027
Folate, DFE	µg	85	24	12
Vitamin A, RAE	µg	146	41	20
Vitamin A, IU	IU	2917	817	408
Vitamin K (phylloquinone)	µg	1140	319.2	159.6
Fatty acids, total saturated	g	0.091	0.025	0.013
Fatty acids, total monounsaturated	g	0.076	0.021	0.011
Fatty acids, total polyunsaturated	g	0.147	0.041	0.021

Source: USDA Nutrient Database

Nutrition in Cooked Amaranth Leaves (boiled, drained, without salt)

Nutrient	Unit	Value per 100g	1.0"cup"132.0g
Water	g	91.49	120.77
Energy	kcal	21	28
Protein	g	2.11	2.79
Total lipid (fat)	g	0.18	0.24
Carbohydrate, by difference	g	4.11	5.43
Calcium, Ca	mg	209	276
Iron, Fe	mg	2.26	2.98
Magnesium, Mg	mg	55	73
Phosphorus, P	mg	72	95
Potassium, K	mg	641	846
Sodium, Na	mg	21	28
Zinc, Zn	mg	0.88	1.16
Vitamin C, total ascorbic acid	mg	41.1	54.3
Thiamin	mg	0.02	0.026
Riboflavin	mg	0.134	0.177
Niacin	mg	0.559	0.738
Vitamin B-6	mg	0.177	0.234
Folate, DFE	µg	57	75
Vitamin B-12	µg	0	0
Vitamin A, RAE	µg	139	183
Vitamin A, IU	IU	2770	3656
Vitamin D (D2 + D3)	µg	0	0
Vitamin D	IU	0	0
Fatty acids, total saturated	g	0.05	0.066
Fatty acids, total monounsaturated	g	0.041	0.054
Fatty acids, total polyunsaturated	g	0.08	0.106
Cholesterol	mg	0	0

Source: USDA Nutrient Database

3

Nutrition in Cooked Amaranth Leaves (boiled, drained, with salt)

Nutrient	Unit	Value per 100g	1.0"cup"132.0g
Water	g	91.49	120.77
Energy	kcal	21	28
Protein	g	2.11	2.79
Total lipid (fat)	g	0.18	0.24
Carbohydrate, by difference	g	4.11	5.43
Calcium, Ca	mg	209	276
Iron, Fe	mg	2.26	2.98
Magnesium, Mg	mg	55	73
Phosphorus, P	mg	72	95
Potassium, K	mg	641	846
Sodium, Na	mg	257	339
Zinc, Zn	mg	0.88	1.16
Vitamin C, total ascorbic acid	mg	41.1	54.3
Thiamin	mg	0.02	0.026
Riboflavin	mg	0.134	0.177
Niacin	mg	0.559	0.738
Vitamin B-6	mg	0.177	0.234
Folate, DFE	µg	57	75
Vitamin B-12	µg	0	0
Vitamin A, RAE	µg	139	183
Vitamin A, IU	IU	2770	3656
Vitamin D (D2 + D3)	µg	0	0
Vitamin D	IU	0	0
Fatty acids, total saturated	g	0.05	0.066
Fatty acids, total monounsaturated	g	0.041	0.054
Fatty acids, total polyunsaturated	g	0.08	0.106
Cholesterol	mg	0	0

Source: USDA Nutrient Database

Arugula

Scientific name of arugula is *Eruca sativa* and it belongs to the family *Brassicaceae*, the cabbage family (syn. Cruciferae). In other words, arugula is a brassica vegetable or a cruciferous vegetable. Arugula is grown for its highly nutritious, pepper-flavoured dark green leaves which are used as a salad vegetable.

Brassica vegetables are biennial in their growing habit but for food purposes they are grown as annuals. Brassica vegetables believed to be originated in the region comprising of Western Europe, the Mediterranean region and the temperate regions of Asia.

Leaves are harvested for consumption while they are tender and young yet ripe and fully grown. Arugula is rich in moisture, dietary fiber and antioxidant vitamins, Vitamin A, Folic acid, Vitamin K and Vitamin C. Since it is rich in antioxidants, consumption of arugula is considered to be good to prevent the life style diseases such as cancer and premature ageing. It is rich in minerals such as iron and copper.

Nutrition in Raw Arugula

Nutrient	Unit	Value per100g	1.0"leaf"2.0 g	0.5"cup"10.0 g
Water	g	91.71	1.83	9.17
Energy	kcal	25	0	2
Protein	g	2.58	0.05	0.26
Total lipid (fat)	g	0.66	0.01	0.07
Carbohydrate, by difference	g	3.65	0.07	0.36
Fiber, total dietary	g	1.6	0	0.2
Sugars, total	g	2.05	0.04	0.2
Calcium, Ca	mg	160	3	16
Iron, Fe	mg	1.46	0.03	0.15
Magnesium, Mg	mg	47	1	5
Phosphorus, P	mg	52	1	5
Potassium, K	mg	369	7	37
Sodium, Na	mg	27	1	3
Zinc, Zn	mg	0.47	0.01	0.05
Vitamin C, total ascorbic acid	mg	15	0.3	1.5
Thiamin	mg	0.044	0.001	0.004
Riboflavin	mg	0.086	0.002	0.009
Niacin	mg	0.305	0.006	0.03
Vitamin B-6	mg	0.073	0.001	0.007
Folate, DFE	µg	97	2	10
Vitamin B-12	µg	0	0	0
Vitamin A, RAE	µg	119	2	12
Vitamin A, IU	IU	2373	47	237
Vitamin E (alpha-tocopherol)	mg	0.43	0.01	0.04
Vitamin K (phylloquinone)	µg	108.6	2.2	10.9
Fatty acids, total saturated	g	0.086	0.002	0.009
Fatty acids, total monounsaturated	g	0.049	0.001	0.005
Fatty acids, total polyunsaturated	g	0.319	0.006	0.032

Source: USDA Nutrient Database

Beet Leaves or Beet Greens

Scientific name of beet leaf is *Beta vulgaris* and it belongs to the family Chenopodiaceae. It is grown as an annual crop for its tender succulent leaves that are used as a highly nutritious leafy vegetable.

Nutrition in Raw Beet Greens per 100 grams of Edible Portion

Nutrient	Unit	Value per100g	1.0"cup "38.0g	1.0"leaf "32.0g	0.5"cup (1" pieces)"19.0g
Water	g	91.02	34.59	29.13	17.29
Energy	kcal	22	8	7	4
Protein	g	2.2	0.84	0.7	0.42
Total lipid (fat)	g	0.13	0.05	0.04	0.02
Carbohydrate, by difference	g	4.33	1.65	1.39	0.82
Fiber, total dietary	g	3.7	1.4	1.2	0.7
Sugars, total	g	0.5	0.19	0.16	0.1
Calcium, Ca	mg	117	44	37	22
Iron, Fe	mg	2.57	0.98	0.82	0.49
Magnesium, Mg	mg	70	27	22	13
Phosphorus, P	mg	41	16	13	8
Potassium, K	mg	762	290	244	145
Sodium, Na	mg	226	86	72	43
Zinc, Zn	mg	0.38	0.14	0.12	0.07
Vitamin C, total ascorbic acid	mg	30	11.4	9.6	5.7

7

Thiamin	mg	0.1	0.038	0.032	0.019
Riboflavin	mg	0.22	0.084	0.07	0.042
Niacin	mg	0.4	0.152	0.128	0.076
Vitamin B-6	mg	0.106	0.04	0.034	0.02
Folate, DFE	µg	15	6	5	3
Vitamin A, RAE	µg	316	120	101	60
Vitamin A, IU	IU	6326	2404	2024	1202
Vitamin E (alpha-tocopherol)	mg	1.5	0.57	0.48	0.28
Vitamin K (phylloquinone)	µg	400	152	128	76
Fatty acids, total saturated	g	0.02	0.008	0.006	0.004
Fatty acids, total monounsaturated	g	0.026	0.01	0.008	0.005
Fatty acids, total polyunsaturated	g	0.046	0.017	0.015	0.009

Source: USDA Nutrient Database

Broccoli Leaves

Scientific name of Broccoli is *Brassica oleracea var. italic.* It is a brassica vegetable and it belongs to the genus Brassica and family Brassicaceae.

Broccoli flower clusters, leaves and leafstalks, and spears are used as vegetables. Here focus is on the use of broccoli leaves as a leafy vegetable. Tender broccoli leaves are used in preparing salads, soups etc. It is a rich source of vitamins and minerals.

It is biennial in growing habit but for food purposes, it is grown as an annual. It is believed to be originated in the region comprising of Western Europe, the Mediterranean region and the temperate regions of Asia.

Nutrition in Raw Broccoli Leaves

Nutrient	Unit	Value per 100g
Water	g	90.69
Energy	kcal	28
Protein	g	2.98
Total lipid (fat)	g	0.35
Carbohydrate, by difference	g	5.24
Calcium, Ca	mg	48
Iron, Fe	mg	0.88
Magnesium, Mg	mg	25
Phosphorus, P	mg	66
Potassium, K	mg	325
Sodium, Na	mg	27
Zinc, Zn	mg	0.4
Vitamin C, total ascorbic acid	mg	93.2
Thiamin	mg	0.065
Riboflavin	mg	0.119
Niacin	mg	0.638
Vitamin B-6	mg	0.159
Folate, DFE	µg	71
Vitamin B-12	µg	0
Vitamin A, RAE	µg	800
Vitamin A, IU	IU	16000
Vitamin D (D2 + D3)	µg	0
Vitamin D	IU	0
Fatty acids, total saturated	g	0.054
Fatty acids, total monounsaturated	g	0.024
Fatty acids, total polyunsaturated	g	0.167
Cholesterol	mg	0

Source: USDA Nutrient Database

Collard Greens

Scientific name of collard greens is *Brassica oleracea cv. acephala*. It is a brassica vegetable and it belongs to the genus Brassica and family Brassicaceae, the mustard family. Collard green is a popular brassica leafy vegetable. It is biennial in growing habit but for food purposes, it is grown as an annual. It is believed to be originated in the region comprising of Western Europe, the Mediterranean region and the temperate regions of Asia.

Collard greens are mainly grown for its thick, highly nutritious leaves. Collard leaves are slightly bitter in taste when consumed in its raw form, especially as an ingredient in salads. Collard greens may be cooked as stir-fries and may be used in soups and stews.

Nutrition in Raw Collards

Nutrient	Unit	Value per100g	1.0"cup, chopped"36.0g
Water	g	89.62	32.26
Energy	kcal	32	12
Protein	g	3.02	1.09
Total lipid (fat)	g	0.61	0.22
Carbohydrate, by difference	g	5.42	1.95
Fiber, total dietary	g	4	1.4
Sugars, total	g	0.46	0.17
Calcium, Ca	mg	232	84
Iron, Fe	mg	0.47	0.17
Magnesium, Mg	mg	27	10
Phosphorus, P	mg	25	9
Potassium, K	mg	213	77
Sodium, Na	mg	17	6
Zinc, Zn	mg	0.21	0.08
Vitamin C, total ascorbic acid	mg	35.3	12.7

Thiamin	mg	0.054	0.019
Riboflavin	mg	0.13	0.047
Niacin	mg	0.742	0.267
Vitamin B-6	mg	0.165	0.059
Folate, DFE	Âµg	129	46
Vitamin B-12	Âµg	0	0
Vitamin A, RAE	Âµg	251	90
Vitamin A, IU	IU	5019	1807
Vitamin E (alpha-tocopherol)	mg	2.26	0.81
Vitamin D (D2 + D3)	Âµg	0	0
Vitamin D	IU	0	0
Vitamin K (phylloquinone)	Âµg	437.1	157.4
Fatty acids, total saturated	g	0.055	0.02
Fatty acids, total monounsaturated	g	0.03	0.011
Fatty acids, total polyunsaturated	g	0.201	0.072
Cholesterol	mg	0	0
Caffeine	mg	0	0

Source: USDA Nutrient Database

Nutrition in Cooked Collards (boiled, drained, without salt)

Nutrient	Unit	Value per100g	1.0"cup, chopped"190.0g
Water	g	90.18	171.34
Energy	kcal	33	63
Protein	g	2.71	5.15
Total lipid (fat)	g	0.72	1.37
Carbohydrate, by difference	g	5.65	10.74
Fiber, total dietary	g	4	7.6
Sugars, total	g	0.4	0.76
Calcium, Ca	mg	141	268
Iron, Fe	mg	1.13	2.15
Magnesium, Mg	mg	21	40
Phosphorus, P	mg	32	61
Potassium, K	mg	117	222
Sodium, Na	mg	15	28
Zinc, Zn	mg	0.23	0.44
Vitamin C, total ascorbic acid	mg	18.2	34.6
Thiamin	mg	0.04	0.076
Riboflavin	mg	0.106	0.201
Niacin	mg	0.575	1.092
Vitamin B-6	mg	0.128	0.243
Folate, DFE	µg	16	30
Vitamin B-12	µg	0	0
Vitamin A, RAE	µg	380	722
Vitamin A, IU	IU	7600	14440
Vitamin E (alpha-tocopherol)	mg	0.88	1.67
Vitamin D	IU	0	0
Vitamin K (phylloquinone)	µg	406.6	772.5
Fatty acids, total saturated	g	0.047	0.089
Fatty acids, total monounsaturated	g	0.026	0.049
Fatty acids, total polyunsaturated	g	0.173	0.329
Cholesterol	mg	0	0

Source: USDA Nutrient Database

13

Nutrition in Frozen Collards (chopped, unprepared)

Nutrient	Unit	Value per100g	0.33"package (10 oz)"95.0g	1.0"package (10 oz)"284.0g	1.0"package (3 lb)"1361.0g
Water	g	89.53	85.05	254.27	1218.5
Energy	kcal	33	31	94	449
Protein	g	2.69	2.56	7.64	36.61
Total lipid (fat)	g	0.37	0.35	1.05	5.04
Carbohydrate, by difference	g	6.46	6.14	18.35	87.92
Fiber, total dietary	g	3.6	3.4	10.2	49
Calcium, Ca	mg	201	191	571	2736
Iron, Fe	mg	1.07	1.02	3.04	14.56
Magnesium, Mg	mg	29	28	82	395
Phosphorus, P	mg	27	26	77	367
Potassium, K	mg	253	240	719	3443
Sodium, Na	mg	48	46	136	653
Zinc, Zn	mg	0.26	0.25	0.74	3.54
Vitamin C, total ascorbic acid	mg	40	38	113.6	544.4
Thiamin	mg	0.05	0.048	0.142	0.68
Riboflavin	mg	0.11	0.104	0.312	1.497
Niacin	mg	0.641	0.609	1.82	8.724
Vitamin B-6	mg	0.115	0.109	0.327	1.565
Folate, DFE	Aµg	73	69	207	994
Vitamin A, RAE	Aµg	459	436	1304	6247
Vitamin A, IU	IU	9183	8724	26080	124981
Fatty acids, total saturated	g	0.048	0.046	0.136	0.653
Fatty acids, total monounsaturated	g	0.027	0.026	0.077	0.367
Fatty acids, total polyunsaturated	g	0.178	0.169	0.506	2.423

Source: USDA Nutrient Database

Nutrition in Frozen Collards (chopped, cooked, boiled, drained, without salt)

Nutrient	Unit	Value per100g	1.0"cup, chopped"170.0g
Water	g	88.47	150.4
Energy	kcal	36	61
Protein	g	2.97	5.05
Total lipid (fat)	g	0.41	0.7
Carbohydrate, by difference	g	7.1	12.07
Fiber, total dietary	g	2.8	4.8
Sugars, total	g	0.57	0.97
Calcium, Ca	mg	210	357
Iron, Fe	mg	1.12	1.9
Magnesium, Mg	mg	30	51
Phosphorus, P	mg	27	46
Potassium, K	mg	251	427
Sodium, Na	mg	50	85
Zinc, Zn	mg	0.27	0.46
Vitamin C, total ascorbic acid	mg	26.4	44.9
Thiamin	mg	0.047	0.08
Riboflavin	mg	0.115	0.196
Niacin	mg	0.635	1.08
Vitamin B-6	mg	0.114	0.194
Folate, DFE	µg	76	129
Vitamin B-12	µg	0	0
Vitamin A, RAE	µg	575	978
Vitamin A, IU	IU	11493	19538
Vitamin E (alpha-tocopherol)	mg	1.25	2.12
Vitamin K (phylloquinone)	µg	623.2	1059.4
Fatty acids, total saturated	g	0.06	0.102
Fatty acids, total monounsaturated	g	0.02	0.034
Fatty acids, total polyunsaturated	g	0.21	0.357
Cholesterol	mg	0	0
Caffeine	mg	0	0

Source: USDA Nutrient Database

Cress or Garden Cress

Scientific name of garden cress is *Lipidium sativum* and it belongs to the family Brassicaceae. It is grown for its edible leaves which are nutritious and with a tangy flavour. Garden cress is used as an ingredient in salads, soups and sandwiches.

Nutrition in Raw Garden Cress

Nutrient	Unit	Value per100g	1.0"cup"50.0 g	1.0"sprig"1.0 g
Proximates				
Water	g	89.4	44.7	0.89
Energy	kcal	32	16	0
Protein	g	2.6	1.3	0.03
Total lipid (fat)	g	0.7	0.35	0.01
Carbohydrate, by difference	g	5.5	2.75	0.06
Fiber, total dietary	g	1.1	0.6	0
Sugars, total	g	4.4	2.2	0.04
Minerals				
Calcium, Ca	mg	81	40	1
Iron, Fe	mg	1.3	0.65	0.01
Magnesium, Mg	mg	38	19	0
Phosphorus, P	mg	76	38	1
Potassium, K	mg	606	303	6
Sodium, Na	mg	14	7	0
Zinc, Zn	mg	0.23	0.12	0
Vitamins				
Vitamin C, total ascorbic acid	mg	69	34.5	0.7
Thiamin	mg	0.08	0.04	0.001
Riboflavin	mg	0.26	0.13	0.003
Niacin	mg	1	0.5	0.01
Vitamin B-6	mg	0.247	0.124	0.002

Folate, DFE	Âμg	80	40	1
Vitamin B-12	Âμg	0	0	0
Vitamin A, RAE	Âμg	346	173	3
Vitamin A, IU	IU	6917	3458	69
Vitamin E (alpha-tocopherol)	mg	0.7	0.35	0.01
Vitamin D (D2 + D3)	Âμg	0	0	0
Vitamin D	IU	0	0	0
Vitamin K (phylloquinone)	Âμg	541.9	271	5.4
Lipids				
Fatty acids, total saturated	g	0.023	0.012	0
Fatty acids, total monounsaturated	g	0.239	0.12	0.002
Fatty acids, total polyunsaturated	g	0.228	0.114	0.002
Cholesterol	mg	0	0	0
Other				
Caffeine	mg	0	0	0

Source: USDA Nutrient Database

Nutrition in Cooked Garden Cress (boiled, drained, without salt)

Nutrient	Unit	Value per100g	1.0"cup"135.0 g	0.5"cup"68.0 g
Water	g	92.5	124.88	62.9
Energy	kcal	23	31	16
Protein	g	1.9	2.56	1.29
Total lipid (fat)	g	0.6	0.81	0.41
Carbohydrate, by difference	g	3.8	5.13	2.58
Fiber, total dietary	g	0.7	0.9	0.5
Sugars, total	g	3.11	4.2	2.11
Calcium, Ca	mg	61	82	41
Iron, Fe	mg	0.8	1.08	0.54
Magnesium, Mg	mg	26	35	18
Phosphorus, P	mg	48	65	33
Potassium, K	mg	353	477	240
Sodium, Na	mg	8	11	5
Zinc, Zn	mg	0.15	0.2	0.1
Vitamin C, total ascorbic acid	mg	23	31	15.6
Thiamin	mg	0.06	0.081	0.041
Riboflavin	mg	0.16	0.216	0.109
Niacin	mg	0.8	1.08	0.544
Vitamin B-6	mg	0.157	0.212	0.107
Folate, DFE	Âµg	37	50	25
Vitamin B-12	Âµg	0	0	0
Vitamin A, RAE	Âµg	232	313	158
Vitamin A, IU	IU	4649	6276	3161
Vitamin E (alpha-tocopherol)	mg	0.5	0.68	0.34
Vitamin K (phylloquinone)	Âµg	383.4	517.6	260.7
Fatty acids, total saturated	g	0.02	0.027	0.014
Fatty acids, total monounsaturated	g	0.205	0.277	0.139
Fatty acids, total polyunsaturated	g	0.196	0.265	0.133

Source: USDA Nutrient Database

18

Colocasia (Taro) Leaves

Botanical name of taro is *Colocasia esculenta* and it belongs to the family Araceae. Both tubers and leaves of taro are edible. It is believed to be a native of South India and South East Asia.

Taro leaves are cooked in various forms; it may be baked, boiled to make soups and/or may be cooked with coconut, pulses, fish or meat to prepare various dishes.

Taro leaves are low in fatty acids and cholesterol and high in calcium, potassium and other essential minerals. It is a rich source of Vitamin E and Vitamin K.

Nutrition in Raw Taro Leaves

Nutrient	Unit	Value per100g	1.0"cup"28.0g	1.0"leaf (11" x 6-1/2")"10.0g
Proximates				
Water	g	85.66	23.98	8.57
Energy	kcal	42	12	4
Protein	g	4.98	1.39	0.5
Total lipid (fat)	g	0.74	0.21	0.07
Carbohydrate, by difference	g	6.7	1.88	0.67
Fiber, total dietary	g	3.7	1	0.4
Sugars, total	g	3.01	0.84	0.3
Minerals				
Calcium, Ca	mg	107	30	11
Iron, Fe	mg	2.25	0.63	0.22
Magnesium, Mg	mg	45	13	4
Phosphorus, P	mg	60	17	6
Potassium, K	mg	648	181	65
Sodium, Na	mg	3	1	0
Zinc, Zn	mg	0.41	0.11	0.04

Vitamins				
Vitamin C, total ascorbic acid	mg	52	14.6	5.2
Thiamin	mg	0.209	0.059	0.021
Riboflavin	mg	0.456	0.128	0.046
Niacin	mg	1.513	0.424	0.151
Vitamin B-6	mg	0.146	0.041	0.015
Folate, DFE	µg	126	35	13
Vitamin B-12	µg	0	0	0
Vitamin A, RAE	µg	241	67	24
Vitamin A, IU	IU	4825	1351	482
Vitamin E (alpha-tocopherol)	mg	2.02	0.57	0.2
Vitamin D (D2 + D3)	µg	0	0	0
Vitamin D	IU	0	0	0
Vitamin K (phylloquinone)	µg	108.6	30.4	10.9
Lipids				
Fatty acids, total saturated	g	0.151	0.042	0.015
Fatty acids, total monounsaturated	g	0.06	0.017	0.006
Fatty acids, total polyunsaturated	g	0.307	0.086	0.031
Cholesterol	mg	0	0	0
Other				
Caffeine	mg	0	0	0

Source: USDA Nutrient Database

Nutrition in Cooked Taro Leaves (steamed, without salt)

Nutrient	Unit	Value per100g	1.0"cup"145.0g
Water	g	92.15	133.62
Energy	kcal	24	35
Protein	g	2.72	3.94
Total lipid (fat)	g	0.41	0.59
Carbohydrate, by difference	g	4.02	5.83
Fiber, total dietary	g	2	2.9
Calcium, Ca	mg	86	125
Iron, Fe	mg	1.18	1.71
Magnesium, Mg	mg	20	29
Phosphorus, P	mg	27	39
Potassium, K	mg	460	667
Sodium, Na	mg	2	3
Zinc, Zn	mg	0.21	0.3
Vitamin C, total ascorbic acid	mg	35.5	51.5
Thiamin	mg	0.139	0.202
Riboflavin	mg	0.38	0.551
Niacin	mg	1.267	1.837
Vitamin B-6	mg	0.072	0.104
Folate, DFE	µg	48	70
Vitamin B-12	µg	0	0
Vitamin A, RAE	µg	212	307
Vitamin A, IU	IU	4238	6145
Vitamin D (D2 + D3)	µg	0	0
Vitamin D	IU	0	0
Fatty acids, total saturated	g	0.083	0.12
Fatty acids, total monounsaturated	g	0.033	0.048
Fatty acids, total polyunsaturated	g	0.168	0.244
Cholesterol	mg	0	0

Source: USDA Nutrient Database

Nutrition in Cooked Taro Leaves (steamed, with salt)

Nutrient	Unit	Value per100g	1.0"cup"145.0g
Water	g	92.15	133.62
Energy	kcal	24	35
Protein	g	2.72	3.94
Total lipid (fat)	g	0.41	0.59
Carbohydrate, by difference	g	3.89	5.64
Fiber, total dietary	g	2	2.9
Calcium, Ca	mg	86	125
Iron, Fe	mg	1.18	1.71
Magnesium, Mg	mg	20	29
Phosphorus, P	mg	27	39
Potassium, K	mg	460	667
Sodium, Na	mg	238	345
Zinc, Zn	mg	0.21	0.3
Vitamin C, total ascorbic acid	mg	35.5	51.5
Thiamin	mg	0.139	0.202
Riboflavin	mg	0.38	0.551
Niacin	mg	1.267	1.837
Vitamin B-6	mg	0.072	0.104
Folate, DFE	µg	48	70
Vitamin B-12	µg	0	0
Vitamin A, RAE	µg	212	307
Vitamin A, IU	IU	4238	6145
Vitamin D (D2 + D3)	µg	0	0
Vitamin D	IU	0	0
Fatty acids, total saturated	g	0.083	0.12
Fatty acids, total monounsaturated	g	0.033	0.048
Fatty acids, total polyunsaturated	g	0.168	0.244
Cholesterol	mg	0	0

Source: USDA Nutrient Database

Curry Leaves

Botanical name of curry leaf plant is *Murraya koenigii*. It belongs to the family Rutaceace, the citrus family. Curry leaf plant has compound leaves with numerous leaflets, sometimes up to 24 leaflets per leaf. Leaves are highly aromatic but slightly bitter in taste. Curry leaf plant is a native of Indian subcontinent where it is found growing in the backyard of almost every household, particularly in South India.

Fresh curry leaves are rich in minerals, vitamins and dietary fibre. Consumption of 100 grams of fresh curry leaves provide a human body approximately 108 kilo calories of energy. Curry leaves are rich in iron (approx. 0.9 milligrams in 100 grams) and hence good for curing iron deficiency. It is rich in minerals like calcium (approx. 830 milligrams in 100 grams) and phosphorus (approx. 57 milligrams in 100 grams) and hence recommended for promoting bone health and oral health.

Fresh curry leaves are rich in beta-carotene (approx. 7560 µg in 100 grams) which is a precursor of Vitamin A. Curry leaves are rich in Vitamin C also. Both vitamin A and vitamin C are antioxidant vitamins which help in reducing oxidative stress and removing free radicals. Other antioxidants present in fresh curry leaves are lutein (27µg/g), alpha tocopherol (592ng/g) and chlorophyll (28mg/g).

Fresh curry leaves are rich in antioxidant vitamin, Vitamin C and antioxidant mineral, Zinc. Beta-carotene is also a major antioxidant plant compound. Vitamin C is water soluble, easily absorbed by the body hence a mighty scavenger of free radicals present in the bodily fluids including blood. Antioxidants present in curry leaves save our body cells from free radical damage and oxidative stress.

Nutritional Value of Fresh Curry Leaves per 100 gram

Nutritional value of fresh curry leaves per 100 gram of edible portion is given below.

Parameters	Value
Moisture	63.8 gm
Protein	6.1 gm
Fat	1.0 gm
Minerals	4.0 gm
Fibre	6.4 gm
Carbohydrates	18.7 gm
Energy	108.0 K cal
Calcium	830.0 mg
Phosphorus	57.0 mg
Iron	0.93 mg
Vitamins	
Carotene	7560 μg
Thiamine	0.080 mg
Riboflavin	0.210 mg
Niacin	2.300 mg
Folic Acid (Free)	23.500 μg
Folic Acid (Total)	93.900 μg
Vitamin C	4 mg
Minerals	
Magnesium	44 mg
Copper	0.100 mg
Manganese	0.150 mg
Zinc	0.200 mg
Chromium	0.006 mg
Sulphur	81 mg
Chlorine	198 mg
Oxalic Acid	132 mg
Phytin Phosphorus	35 mg

Source: Spices Board, India

Curry leaves and curry leaf essential oil are used for culinary purposes, medicinal purposes and as an ingredient in the production of cosmetics such as soaps and deodorants.

Fresh curry leaves are an essential spice ingredient in many South Indian food preparations including curries and pickles. Curry leaves are used in small quantities to add its distinctive flavor and aroma to the food. The essential oil present in the leaves is released only when leaves are fried in the oil or ghee. So the first step in any food preparation that uses curry leaves is to add small quantities of fresh leaves in heated oil or ghee and then fry it for some time so that aroma and flavor is released into the oil completely.

Curry leaf plant is an ancient Indian plant that has extensively been used in Indian traditional medicines since time immemorial. Mainly fresh leaves, bark and roots of curry leaf plant and curry leaf essential oil are used in medicinal preparations.

Approximately 400 to 500 grams of fresh leaves is obtained per plant per year in three to four pickings. Freshly harvested curry leaves can be stored at room temperature up to one week. Long term storage is possible by freezing and drying. In drying, air drying and oven-drying may be practiced. However curry leaves lose their delicate fragrance soon after drying.

Chrysanthemum Leaves (Edible Chrysanthemum)

Botanical name of edible chrysanthemum is *Glebionis coronaria* (syn. *Chrysanthemum coronarium*) and it belongs to aster family i.e. Asteraceae. Edible chrysanthemum is believed to be originated in the Mediterranean region and East Asia.

Edible chrysanthemum or chrysanthemum greens is also known as garland chrysanthemum, crown daisy, and Japanese green. Edible chrysanthemum is an annual herbaceous plant which produces fragrant yellow flowers upon maturity. Edible leaves are harvested at its tender stage which is well ahead of its flowering time.

Edible chrysanthemum leaves are rich in dietary fiber at 3g/100 g and minerals with calcium at 117mg/100 g; potassium at 567 mg/100 g; and sodium at 118 mg/100 g. It is also rich in vitamins with the presence Vitamin A and Vitamin C in high concentrations.

Chrysanthemum greens may be used in the preparation of soups and stews or may be added as an ingredient in the preparation of omelettes and other egg preparations. It may also be stir-fried or steamed as a leafy vegetable.

Nutrition in Raw Chrysanthemum Leaves

Nutrient	Unit	Value per100g	1.0"cup, chopped"51.0g	1.0"leaf"18.0g
Water	g	91.4	46.61	16.45
Energy	kcal	24	12	4
Protein	g	3.36	1.71	0.6
Total lipid (fat)	g	0.56	0.29	0.1
Carbohydrate, by difference	g	3.01	1.54	0.54
Fiber, total dietary	g	3	1.5	0.5
Calcium, Ca	mg	117	60	21
Iron, Fe	mg	2.3	1.17	0.41
Magnesium, Mg	mg	32	16	6
Phosphorus, P	mg	54	28	10
Potassium, K	mg	567	289	102
Sodium, Na	mg	118	60	21
Zinc, Zn	mg	0.71	0.36	0.13
Vitamin C, total ascorbic acid	mg	1.4	0.7	0.3
Thiamin	mg	0.13	0.066	0.023
Riboflavin	mg	0.144	0.073	0.026
Niacin	mg	0.531	0.271	0.096
Vitamin B-6	mg	0.176	0.09	0.032
Folate, DFE	µg	177	90	32
Vitamin B-12	µg	0	0	0
Vitamin A, RAE	µg	94	48	17
Vitamin A, IU	IU	1870	954	337
Vitamin D (D2 + D3)	µg	0	0	0
Vitamin D	IU	0	0	0
Cholesterol	mg	0	0	0

Source: USDA Nutrient Database

27

Drumstick (Moringa) Leaves

Scientific name of moringa is *Moringa oleifera*. It is a multipurpose tree and leaves of which are used a leafy vegetable. Moringa leaves can be used as a raw leafy vegetable just like spinach. Fresh Moringa leaf juice is also a highly nutritious diet. As per USDA Nutrient Database, consumption of 100 gram of edible portion of fresh Moringa leaves provides a human body with approx. 64 kilo calories of energy and almost same amount of protein of eggs and yoghurt. Similarly, Moringa leaves contain more Calcium than that of buffalo milk; more Iron than that of Spinach, same amount of Potassium of raw bananas, same amount of Vitamin C of navel oranges and almost half of Vitamin A of carrots.

A comparative study of nutrition in Moringa leaves against that of foods considered as highest sources of various nutrients is given below:

Nutrient per 100 g edible portion	Moringa leaves	Foods considered as one of the highest sources of this nutrient (per 100 g of edible portion)
Protein	9.4 g	Eggs - 12.56 g Yoghurt - 11.12 g
Calcium	185 mg	Buffalo Milk - 169 mg
Iron	4 mg	Spinach - 2.71mg
Potassium	337 mg	Raw Bananas - 358 mg
Vitamin C	51.7 mg	Navel Oranges - 59 mg
Vitamin A	7564 IU	Carrots - 16706 IU

Source: USDA Nutrient Database

Moringa leaves are also rich sources of magnesium and phosphorus and Vitamin B-complex. A description of various nutrients present in fresh Moringa leaves is given below:

Nutrition in Raw (fresh) Drumstick Leaves

Nutrient	Unit	Value per 100g
Proximates		
Water	g	78.66
Energy	kcal	64
Protein	g	9.4
Total lipid (fat)	g	1.4
Carbohydrate, by difference	g	8.28
Fiber, total dietary	g	2
Minerals		
Calcium, Ca	mg	185
Iron, Fe	mg	4
Magnesium, Mg	mg	147
Phosphorus, P	mg	112
Potassium, K	mg	337
Sodium, Na	mg	9
Zinc, Zn	mg	0.6
Vitamins		
Vitamin C, total ascorbic acid	mg	51.7
Thiamin	mg	0.257
Riboflavin	mg	0.66
Niacin	mg	2.22
Vitamin B-6	mg	1.2
Folate, DFE	µg	40
Vitamin B-12	µg	0
Vitamin A, RAE	µg	378
Vitamin A, IU	IU	7564
Vitamin D (D2 + D3)	µg	0
Vitamin D	IU	0
Lipids		
Cholesterol	mg	0

Source: USDA Nutrient Database

29

Boiled Moringa Leaves as a Leafy Vegetable

Leaves are normally cooked by steaming or boiling to preserve its nutrients. Overcooking (above 140 degrees Fahrenheit) needs to be avoided as it may result in loss of some nutrients. Boiling with salt increases sodium content of the food. A description of various nutrients present in boiled Moringa leaves is given below:

Nutrition in Drumstick Leaves, Cooked, Boiled, and Drained

Nutrient	Unit	Value per 100g	
		WITHOUT SALT	WITH SALT
Water	g	81.65	81.65
Energy	kcal	60	60
Protein	g	5.27	5.27
Total lipid (fat)	g	0.93	0.93
Carbohydrate, by difference	g	11.15	11.15
Fiber, total dietary	g	2	2
Sugars, total	g	1	1
Calcium, Ca	mg	151	151
Iron, Fe	mg	2.32	2.32
Magnesium, Mg	mg	151	151
Phosphorus, P	mg	67	67
Potassium, K	mg	344	344
Sodium, Na	mg	9	245
Zinc, Zn	mg	0.49	0.49
Vitamin C, total ascorbic acid	mg	31	31
Thiamin	mg	0.222	0.222
Riboflavin	mg	0.509	0.509
Niacin	mg	1.995	1.995
Vitamin B-6	mg	0.929	0.929
Folate, DFE	µg	23	23
Vitamin B-12	µg	0	0
Vitamin A, RAE	µg	351	351
Vitamin A, IU	IU	7013	7013
Vitamin E (alpha-tocopherol)	mg	0.1	0.1
Vitamin D (D2 + D3)	µg	0	0
Vitamin D	IU	0	0
Vitamin K (phylloquinone)	µg	108	108
Fatty acids, total saturated	G	0.152	0
Fatty acids, total monounsaturated	G	0.473	0
Fatty acids, total polyunsaturated	G	0.015	0
Cholesterol	Mg	0	0
Caffeine	Mg	0	0

Source: USDA Nutrient Database

Dandelion Greens

Scientific name of dandelion is *Taraxacum officinale* and it belongs to the family Asteraceae, the chrysanthemum family. Fresh dandelion leaves are used as a leafy vegetable and it is considered as a multivitamin green. It is high in calcium, rich in iron, low in calories, and loaded with lots of antioxidants.

Nutrition in Raw Dandelion Greens

Nutrient	Unit	Value per100g	1.0"cup, chopped"55.0g
Water	g	85.6	47.08
Energy	kcal	45	25
Protein	g	2.7	1.48
Total lipid (fat)	g	0.7	0.38
Carbohydrate, by difference	g	9.2	5.06
Fiber, total dietary	g	3.5	1.9
Sugars, total	g	0.71	0.39
Calcium, Ca	mg	187	103
Iron, Fe	mg	3.1	1.7
Magnesium, Mg	mg	36	20
Phosphorus, P	mg	66	36
Potassium, K	mg	397	218
Sodium, Na	mg	76	42
Zinc, Zn	mg	0.41	0.23
Vitamin C, total ascorbic acid	mg	35	19.2
Thiamin	mg	0.19	0.104
Riboflavin	mg	0.26	0.143
Niacin	mg	0.806	0.443
Vitamin B-6	mg	0.251	0.138

Folate, DFE	Âμg	27	15
Vitamin A, RAE	Âμg	508	279
Vitamin A, IU	IU	10161	5589
Vitamin E (alpha-tocopherol)	mg	3.44	1.89
Vitamin K (phylloquinone)	Âμg	778.4	428.1
Fatty acids, total saturated	g	0.17	0.094
Fatty acids, total monounsaturated	g	0.014	0.008
Fatty acids, total polyunsaturated	g	0.306	0.168

Source: USDA Nutrient Database

Nutrition in Cooked Dandelion greens (boiled, drained, without salt)

Nutrient	Unit	Value per100g	1.0"cup, chopped"105.0g
Water	g	89.8	94.29
Energy	kcal	33	35
Protein	g	2	2.1
Total lipid (fat)	g	0.6	0.63
Carbohydrate, by difference	g	6.4	6.72
Fiber, total dietary	g	2.9	3
Sugars, total	g	0.5	0.52
Calcium, Ca	mg	140	147
Iron, Fe	mg	1.8	1.89
Magnesium, Mg	mg	24	25
Phosphorus, P	mg	42	44
Potassium, K	mg	232	244
Sodium, Na	mg	44	46
Zinc, Zn	mg	0.28	0.29
Vitamin C, total ascorbic acid	mg	18	18.9
Thiamin	mg	0.13	0.136
Riboflavin	mg	0.175	0.184
Niacin	mg	0.514	0.54
Vitamin B-6	mg	0.16	0.168
Folate, DFE	Âµg	13	14
Vitamin A, RAE	Âµg	342	359
Vitamin A, IU	IU	6837	7179
Vitamin E (alpha-tocopherol)	mg	2.44	2.56
Vitamin K (phylloquinone)	Âµg	551.4	579
Fatty acids, total saturated	g	0.146	0.153
Fatty acids, total monounsaturated	g	0.012	0.013
Fatty acids, total polyunsaturated	g	0.262	0.275

Source: USDA Nutrient Database

Nutrition in Cooked Dandelion Greens (boiled, drained, with salt)

Nutrient	Unit	Value per100g	1.0"cup, chopped"105.0g
Water	g	89.8	94.29
Energy	kcal	33	35
Protein	g	2	2.1
Total lipid (fat)	g	0.6	0.63
Carbohydrate, by difference	g	6.4	6.72
Fiber, total dietary	g	2.9	3
Sugars, total	g	1.62	1.7
Calcium, Ca	mg	140	147
Iron, Fe	mg	1.8	1.89
Magnesium, Mg	mg	24	25
Phosphorus, P	mg	42	44
Potassium, K	mg	232	244
Sodium, Na	mg	280	294
Zinc, Zn	mg	0.28	0.29
Vitamin C, total ascorbic acid	mg	18	18.9
Thiamin	mg	0.13	0.136
Riboflavin	mg	0.175	0.184
Niacin	mg	0.514	0.54
Vitamin B-6	mg	0.16	0.168
Folate, DFE	µg	13	14
Vitamin A, RAE	µg	727	763
Vitamin A, IU	IU	14544	15271
Vitamin E (alpha-tocopherol)	mg	0.6	0.63
Vitamin K (phylloquinone)	µg	358.9	376.8

Source: USDA Nutrient Database

34

Docks and Sorrels

Scientific name of sorrel is *Rumex acetosa*. Scientific name of dock is *Rumex patientia*. Docks and sorrels belong to the family Polygonaceae.

Docks and sorrels are perennial herbaceous plants that are believed to be originated in British Isles. These plants are grown for its large, nutritious leaves which are a rich source of minerals and vitamins.

Nutrition in Raw Dock

Nutrient	Unit	Value per100g	1.0"cup, chopped"133.0g
Water	g	93	123.69
Energy	kcal	22	29
Protein	g	2	2.66
Total lipid (fat)	g	0.7	0.93
Carbohydrate, by difference	g	3.2	4.26
Fiber, total dietary	g	2.9	3.9
Calcium, Ca	mg	44	59
Iron, Fe	mg	2.4	3.19
Magnesium, Mg	mg	103	137
Phosphorus, P	mg	63	84
Potassium, K	mg	390	519
Sodium, Na	mg	4	5
Zinc, Zn	mg	0.2	0.27
Vitamin C, total ascorbic acid	mg	48	63.8
Thiamin	mg	0.04	0.053
Riboflavin	mg	0.1	0.133
Niacin	mg	0.5	0.665
Vitamin B-6	mg	0.122	0.162
Folate, DFE	µg	13	17
Vitamin B-12	µg	0	0
Vitamin A, RAE	µg	200	266
Vitamin A, IU	IU	4000	5320

Source: USDA Nutrient Database

Nutrition in Cooked Dock (boiled, drained, without salt)

Nutrient	Unit	Value per100g
Proximates		
Water	g	93.6
Energy	kcal	20
Protein	g	1.83
Total lipid (fat)	g	0.64
Carbohydrate, by difference	g	2.93
Fiber, total dietary	g	2.6
Minerals		
Calcium, Ca	mg	38
Iron, Fe	mg	2.08
Magnesium, Mg	mg	89
Phosphorus, P	mg	52
Potassium, K	mg	321
Sodium, Na	mg	3
Zinc, Zn	mg	0.17
Vitamins		
Vitamin C, total ascorbic acid	mg	26.3
Thiamin	mg	0.034
Riboflavin	mg	0.086
Niacin	mg	0.411
Vitamin B-6	mg	0.1
Folate, DFE	µg	8
Vitamin B-12	µg	0
Vitamin A, RAE	µg	174
Vitamin A, IU	IU	3474
Vitamin D (D2 + D3)	µg	0
Vitamin D	IU	0
Lipids		
Cholesterol	mg	0

Source: USDA Nutrient Database

English Spinach or True Spinach

Spinach is a very popular leafy vegetable in many parts of the world. Scientific name of spinach is *Spinacia oleracea* and it belongs to the family Amaranthacea.

Tender and succulent leaves of spinach are used in salad preparations, soups and omelettes. Spinach may be cooked as a main vegetable dish or may be used as a side ingredient along with other vegetables. Spinach is considered as one of the highly nutritious leafy vegetables that are available today for human consumption.

Nutrition in Raw Spinach

Nutrient	Unit	Value per100g	1.0"cup"30.0g	1.0"bunch"340.0g	1.0"leaf"10.0g
Proximates					
Water	g	91.4	27.42	310.76	9.14
Energy	kcal	23	7	78	2
Protein	g	2.86	0.86	9.72	0.29
Total lipid (fat)	g	0.39	0.12	1.33	0.04
Carbohydrate, by difference	g	3.63	1.09	12.34	0.36
Fiber, total dietary	g	2.2	0.7	7.5	0.2
Sugars, total	g	0.42	0.13	1.43	0.04
Minerals					
Calcium, Ca	mg	99	30	337	10
Iron, Fe	mg	2.71	0.81	9.21	0.27
Magnesium, Mg	mg	79	24	269	8
Phosphorus, P	mg	49	15	167	5
Potassium, K	mg	558	167	1897	56
Sodium, Na	mg	79	24	269	8
Zinc, Zn	mg	0.53	0.16	1.8	0.05

Vitamins					
Vitamin C, total ascorbic acid	mg	28.1	8.4	95.5	2.8
Thiamin	mg	0.078	0.023	0.265	0.008
Riboflavin	mg	0.189	0.057	0.643	0.019
Niacin	mg	0.724	0.217	2.462	0.072
Vitamin B-6	mg	0.195	0.058	0.663	0.02
Folate, DFE	Âµg	194	58	660	19
Vitamin B-12	Âµg	0	0	0	0
Vitamin A, RAE	Âµg	469	141	1595	47
Vitamin A, IU	IU	9377	2813	31882	938
Vitamin E (alpha-tocopherol)	mg	2.03	0.61	6.9	0.2
Vitamin D (D2 + D3)	Âµg	0	0	0	0
Vitamin D	IU	0	0	0	0
Vitamin K (phylloquinone)	Âµg	482.9	144.9	1641.9	48.3
Lipids					
Fatty acids, total saturated	g	0.063	0.019	0.214	0.006
Fatty acids, total monounsaturated	g	0.01	0.003	0.034	0.001
Fatty acids, total polyunsaturated	g	0.165	0.05	0.561	0.016
Cholesterol	mg	0	0	0	0
Other					
Caffeine	mg	0	0	0	0

Source: USDA Nutrient Database

Nutrition in Cooked Spinach (boiled, drained, without salt)

Nutrient	Unit	Value per100g	1.0"cup"180.0g
Water	g	91.21	164.18
Energy	kcal	23	41
Protein	g	2.97	5.35
Total lipid (fat)	g	0.26	0.47
Carbohydrate, by difference	g	3.75	6.75
Fiber, total dietary	g	2.4	4.3
Sugars, total	g	0.43	0.77
Calcium, Ca	mg	136	245
Iron, Fe	mg	3.57	6.43
Magnesium, Mg	mg	87	157
Phosphorus, P	mg	56	101
Potassium, K	mg	466	839
Sodium, Na	mg	70	126
Zinc, Zn	mg	0.76	1.37
Vitamin C, total ascorbic acid	mg	9.8	17.6
Thiamin	mg	0.095	0.171
Riboflavin	mg	0.236	0.425
Niacin	mg	0.49	0.882
Vitamin B-6	mg	0.242	0.436
Folate, DFE	µg	146	263
Vitamin A, RAE	µg	524	943
Vitamin A, IU	IU	10481	18866
Vitamin E (alpha-tocopherol)	mg	2.08	3.74
Vitamin K (phylloquinone)	µg	493.6	888.5
Fatty acids, total saturated	g	0.043	0.077
Fatty acids, total monounsaturated	g	0.006	0.011
Fatty acids, total polyunsaturated	g	0.109	0.196
Cholesterol	mg	0	0

Source: USDA Nutrient Database

39

Nutrition in Frozen Spinach (chopped or leaf, unprepared)

Nutrient	Unit	Value per100g	1.0"cup"156.0g	1.0"package (10 oz)"284.0g
Water	g	90.17	140.67	256.08
Energy	kcal	29	45	82
Protein	g	3.63	5.66	10.31
Total lipid (fat)	g	0.57	0.89	1.62
Carbohydrate, by difference	g	4.21	6.57	11.96
Fiber, total dietary	g	2.9	4.5	8.2
Sugars, total	g	0.65	1.01	1.85
Calcium, Ca	mg	129	201	366
Iron, Fe	mg	1.89	2.95	5.37
Magnesium, Mg	mg	75	117	213
Phosphorus, P	mg	49	76	139
Potassium, K	mg	346	540	983
Sodium, Na	mg	74	115	210
Zinc, Zn	mg	0.56	0.87	1.59
Vitamin C, total ascorbic acid	mg	5.5	8.6	15.6
Thiamin	mg	0.094	0.147	0.267
Riboflavin	mg	0.224	0.349	0.636
Niacin	mg	0.507	0.791	1.44
Vitamin B-6	mg	0.172	0.268	0.488
Folate, DFE	Âµg	145	226	412
Vitamin A, RAE	Âµg	586	914	1664
Vitamin A, IU	IU	11726	18293	33302
Vitamin E (alpha-tocopherol)	mg	2.9	4.52	8.24
Vitamin K (phylloquinone)	Âµg	372	580.3	1056.5
Fatty acids, total saturated	g	0.041	0.064	0.116
Fatty acids, total monounsaturated	g	0	0	0
Fatty acids, total polyunsaturated	g	0.082	0.128	0.233
Cholesterol	mg	0	0	0

Source: USDA Nutrient Database

Nutrition in Frozen Spinach chopped or leaf, cooked, boiled, drained, without salt)

Nutrient	Unit	Value per100g	0.5"cup"9 5.0g	1.0"package (10 oz) yields"220.0g
Water	g	88.94	84.49	195.67
Energy	kcal	34	32	75
Protein	g	4.01	3.81	8.82
Total lipid (fat)	g	0.87	0.83	1.91
Carbohydrate, by difference	g	4.8	4.56	10.56
Fiber, total dietary	g	3.7	3.5	8.1
Sugars, total	g	0.51	0.48	1.12
Calcium, Ca	mg	153	145	337
Iron, Fe	mg	1.96	1.86	4.31
Magnesium, Mg	mg	82	78	180
Phosphorus, P	mg	50	48	110
Potassium, K	mg	302	287	664
Sodium, Na	mg	97	92	213
Zinc, Zn	mg	0.49	0.47	1.08
Vitamin C, total ascorbic acid	mg	2.2	2.1	4.8
Thiamin	mg	0.078	0.074	0.172
Riboflavin	mg	0.176	0.167	0.387
Niacin	mg	0.439	0.417	0.966
Vitamin B-6	mg	0.136	0.129	0.299
Folate, DFE	Âµg	121	115	266
Vitamin A, RAE	Âµg	603	573	1327
Vitamin A, IU	IU	12061	11458	26534
Vitamin E (alpha-tocopherol)	mg	3.54	3.36	7.79
Vitamin K (phylloquinone)	Âµg	540.7	513.7	1189.5
Fatty acids, total saturated	g	0.157	0.149	0.345
Fatty acids, total monounsaturated	g	0	0	0
Fatty acids, total polyunsaturated	g	0.371	0.352	0.816
Cholesterol	mg	0	0	0

Source: USDA Nutrient Database

41

Endive

Scientific name of endive is *Cichorium endivia* and it belongs to the family Asteraceae, the Daisy family. Endive is mainly grown for its edible leaves which may be consumed in its raw or cooked form.

Raw endive leaves are used in the preparation of green salads and sandwiches while cooked leaves are used as a vegetable dish. Chopped leaves may be used in the preparation of soups, stews, and spicy omelettes. It is a highly nutritious leafy vegetable loaded with lots of vitamins, particularly Vitamin A and Vitamin K, and minerals and dietary fiber.

Nutrition in Raw Endive

Nutrient	Unit	Value per100g	0.5"cup, chopped"25.0g	1.0"head"513.0g
Proximates				
Water	g	93.79	23.45	481.14
Energy	kcal	17	4	87
Protein	g	1.25	0.31	6.41
Total lipid (fat)	g	0.2	0.05	1.03
Carbohydrate, by difference	g	3.35	0.84	17.19
Fiber, total dietary	g	3.1	0.8	15.9
Sugars, total	g	0.25	0.06	1.28
Minerals				
Calcium, Ca	mg	52	13	267
Iron, Fe	mg	0.83	0.21	4.26
Magnesium, Mg	mg	15	4	77
Phosphorus, P	mg	28	7	144
Potassium, K	mg	314	78	1611
Sodium, Na	mg	22	6	113
Zinc, Zn	mg	0.79	0.2	4.05

Vitamins				
Vitamin C, total ascorbic acid	mg	6.5	1.6	33.3
Thiamin	mg	0.08	0.02	0.41
Riboflavin	mg	0.075	0.019	0.385
Niacin	mg	0.4	0.1	2.052
Vitamin B-6	mg	0.02	0.005	0.103
Folate, DFE	Âµg	142	36	728
Vitamin B-12	Âµg	0	0	0
Vitamin A, RAE	Âµg	108	27	554
Vitamin A, IU	IU	2167	542	11117
Vitamin E (alpha-tocopherol)	mg	0.44	0.11	2.26
Vitamin D (D2 + D3)	Âµg	0	0	0
Vitamin D	IU	0	0	0
Vitamin K (phylloquinone)	Âµg	231	57.8	1185
Lipids				
Fatty acids, total saturated	g	0.048	0.012	0.246
Fatty acids, total monounsaturated	g	0.004	0.001	0.021
Fatty acids, total polyunsaturated	g	0.087	0.022	0.446
Cholesterol	mg	0	0	0
Caffeine	mg	0	0	0

Source: USDA Nutrient Database

Fenugreek Leaves or Greek Hay

Scientific name of fenugreek is *Trigonella foenum-graecum* and it belongs to the family *Fabaceae*. It is believed to be originated in Ethiopian region in Africa and Europe.

Tender young fenugreek leaves are used as a leafy vegetable. Consumption of fenugreek leaves aids in alleviating stomach problems such as indigestion and constipation, and stimulates spleen and liver functions. Fenugreek leaves are rich in vitamins, minerals, antioxidants, and dietary fiber.

Nutrition in Raw Fenugreek Leaves per 100 gram of Edible Portion

Nutrient	Value per 100 g
Moisture	86.1 g
Carbohydrates	6.0 g
Protein	4.4 g
Fat	0.9 g
Fiber	1.1 g
Calcium	395 mg
Oxalic acid	13 mg
Magnesium	67 mg
Phosphorus	51 mg
Sodium	76.1 mg
Potassium	31 mg
Sulphur	167 mg
Iron	17.2 mg
Copper	0.26 mg
Chlorine	165 mg
Thiamine	0.05 mg
Riboflavin	0.15 mg
Nicotinic acid	0.7 mg
Vitamin A	6,450 IU
Vitamin C	54 mg
Total energy	49 kcal

Source: Vegetables by Choudhury

Fireweed Leaves

Scientific name of fireweed is *Chamerion angustifolium*. It is also known as Willow-herb. Fireweed is a perennial herbaceous plant belonging to the family Onagraceae. Fireweed leaves may be consumed in its raw form as an ingredient in vegetable salads.

Nutrition in Raw Fireweed Leaves

Nutrient	Unit	Value per100g	1.0"cup, chopped"23.0g	1.0"plant"22.0g
Water	g	70.78	16.28	15.57
Energy	kcal	103	24	23
Protein	g	4.71	1.08	1.04
Total lipid (fat)	g	2.75	0.63	0.6
Carbohydrate, by difference	g	19.22	4.42	4.23
Fiber, total dietary	g	10.6	2.4	2.3
Calcium, Ca	mg	429	99	94
Iron, Fe	mg	2.4	0.55	0.53
Magnesium, Mg	mg	156	36	34
Phosphorus, P	mg	108	25	24
Potassium, K	mg	494	114	109
Sodium, Na	mg	34	8	7
Zinc, Zn	mg	2.66	0.61	0.59
Vitamin C, total ascorbic acid	mg	2.2	0.5	0.5
Thiamin	mg	0.033	0.008	0.007
Riboflavin	mg	0.137	0.032	0.03
Niacin	mg	4.674	1.075	1.028
Vitamin B-6	mg	0.632	0.145	0.139
Folate, DFE	µg	112	26	25
Vitamin A, RAE	µg	180	41	40
Vitamin A, IU	IU	3598	828	792

Source: USDA Nutrient Database

Grape Leaves

Scientific name of grape vine is *Vitis vinefera* and it belongs to the family Vitaceae. Freshly harvested young tender leaves of grape vines may be used as an ingredient in the preparation of various food dishes. In some countries fresh grape leaves are stuffed with a spicy rice and meat mixture and then steamed or boiled until all the ingredients are cooked properly. Fresh grape leaves may be preserved for a long time in a brine solution containing water, salt, and citric acid, and preservatives such as sodium benzoate, potassium sorbate, and sodium bisulfite.

Nutrition in Raw Grape Leaves

Nutrient	Unit	Value per100g	1.0"cup"14.0g	1.0"leaf"3.0g
Proximates				
Water	g	73.32	10.26	2.2
Energy	kcal	93	13	3
Protein	g	5.6	0.78	0.17
Total lipid (fat)	g	2.12	0.3	0.06
Carbohydrate, by difference	g	17.31	2.42	0.52
Fiber, total dietary	g	11	1.5	0.3
Sugars, total	g	6.3	0.88	0.19
Minerals				
Calcium, Ca	mg	363	51	11
Iron, Fe	mg	2.63	0.37	0.08
Magnesium, Mg	mg	95	13	3
Phosphorus, P	mg	91	13	3
Potassium, K	mg	272	38	8
Sodium, Na	mg	9	1	0
Zinc, Zn	mg	0.67	0.09	0.02
Vitamins				

Vitamin C, total ascorbic acid	mg	11.1	1.6	0.3
Thiamin	mg	0.04	0.006	0.001
Riboflavin	mg	0.354	0.05	0.011
Niacin	mg	2.362	0.331	0.071
Vitamin B-6	mg	0.4	0.056	0.012
Folate, DFE	µg	83	12	2
Vitamin B-12	µg	0	0	0
Vitamin A, RAE	µg	1376	193	41
Vitamin A, IU	IU	27521	3853	826
Vitamin E (alpha-tocopherol)	mg	2	0.28	0.06
Vitamin D (D2 + D3)	µg	0	0	0
Vitamin D	IU	0	0	0
Vitamin K (phylloquinone)	µg	108.6	15.2	3.3
Lipids				
Fatty acids, total saturated	g	0.336	0.047	0.01
Fatty acids, total monounsaturated	g	0.081	0.011	0.002
Fatty acids, total polyunsaturated	g	1.065	0.149	0.032
Cholesterol	mg	0	0	0
Other				
Caffeine	mg	0	0	0

Source: USDA Nutrient Database

Kale Leaves

Scientific name of Kale is *Brassica oleracea var. acephala*. It is a specialty Brassica vegetable belonging to family Brassicaceae (Cruciferae), the cabbage family. Kale is a temperate cool season crop which is mainly grown for its edible leaves which may either green or purple (violet) in colour. Kale leaves have a distinct strong flavour and aroma. Kale is also known as borecole. Just like other Brassica vegetables, kale is naturally grown as a biennial but for commercial purposes it is cultivated as an annual vegetable crop. Kale is very easy to grow and it is popular among growers because of its high nutrient value. Kale leaves are rich in minerals, vitamins and antioxidants.

Tender, fresh kale leaves are used in preparing salads. With the addition of its intense flavour, kale leaves make wonderful fresh salads.

Nutrition in Raw (Fresh) Kale Leaves

Nutrient	Unit	Value per100g	1.0"cup, chopped"67.0g
Proximates			
Water	g	84.04	56.31
Energy	kcal	49	33
Protein	g	4.28	2.87
Total lipid (fat)	g	0.93	0.62
Carbohydrate, by difference	g	8.75	5.86
Fiber, total dietary	g	3.6	2.4
Sugars, total	g	2.26	1.51
Minerals			
Calcium, Ca	mg	150	100
Iron, Fe	mg	1.47	0.98
Magnesium, Mg	mg	47	31
Phosphorus, P	mg	92	62

Potassium, K	mg	491	329
Sodium, Na	mg	38	25
Zinc, Zn	mg	0.56	0.38
Vitamins			
Vitamin C, total ascorbic acid	mg	120	80.4
Thiamin	mg	0.11	0.074
Riboflavin	mg	0.13	0.087
Niacin	mg	1	0.67
Vitamin B-6	mg	0.271	0.182
Folate, DFE	µg	141	94
Vitamin B-12	µg	0	0
Vitamin A, RAE	µg	500	335
Vitamin A, IU	IU	9990	6693
Vitamin E (alpha-tocopherol)	mg	1.54	1.03
Vitamin D (D2 + D3)	µg	0	0
Vitamin D	IU	0	0
Vitamin K (phylloquinone)	µg	704.8	472.2
Lipids			
Fatty acids, total saturated	g	0.091	0.061
Fatty acids, total monounsaturated	g	0.052	0.035
Fatty acids, total polyunsaturated	g	0.338	0.226
Cholesterol	mg	0	0
Other			
Caffeine	mg	0	0

Source: USDA Nutrient Database

Kale leaves freeze well under optimum freezing temperature. Frozen unprepared kale leaves taste sweeter and is more flavourful than unfrozen kale.

Nutrition in Frozen, Unprepared Kale

Nutrient	Unit	Value per100g	0.333"package (10 oz)"94.0g	1.0"package (10 oz)"284.0g
Proximates				
Water	g	91.12	85.65	258.78
Energy	kcal	28	26	80
Protein	g	2.66	2.5	7.55
Total lipid (fat)	g	0.46	0.43	1.31
Carbohydrate, by difference	g	4.9	4.61	13.92
Fiber, total dietary	g	2	1.9	5.7
Minerals				
Calcium, Ca	mg	136	128	386
Iron, Fe	mg	0.93	0.87	2.64
Magnesium, Mg	mg	18	17	51
Phosphorus, P	mg	29	27	82
Potassium, K	mg	333	313	946
Sodium, Na	mg	15	14	43
Zinc, Zn	mg	0.18	0.17	0.51
Vitamins				
Vitamin C, total ascorbic acid	mg	39.3	36.9	111.6
Thiamin	mg	0.056	0.053	0.159
Riboflavin	mg	0.112	0.105	0.318
Niacin	mg	0.698	0.656	1.982
Vitamin B-6	mg	0.09	0.085	0.256
Folate, DFE	µg	17	16	48
Vitamin B-12	µg	0	0	0
Vitamin A, RAE	µg	313	294	889
Vitamin A, IU	IU	6253	5878	17759
Vitamin D (D2 + D3)	µg	0	0	0

Vitamin D	IU	0	0	0
Lipids				
Fatty acids, total saturated	g	0.059	0.055	0.168
Fatty acids, total monounsaturated	g	0.034	0.032	0.097
Fatty acids, total polyunsaturated	g	0.219	0.206	0.622
Cholesterol	mg	0	0	0

Source: USDA Nutrient Database

Most common form of cooking kale is by boiling. It may be boiled with or without salt. For boiling kale leaves without salt, whole leaves are taken together and washed thoroughly to clean it. No need to shake off the extra water. Then washed leaves are placed in a pan and covered before placing the pan on a low flame. Cook the kale leaves for about 2 minutes or until the leaves are wilted and then drain thoroughly before using it.

Nutrition in Cooked Kale (Boiled without salt and Drained)

Nutrient	Unit	Value per100g	1.0"cup, chopped"130.0g
Proximates			
Water	g	91.2	118.56
Energy	kcal	28	36
Protein	g	1.9	2.47
Total lipid (fat)	g	0.4	0.52
Carbohydrate, by difference	g	5.63	7.32
Fiber, total dietary	g	2	2.6
Sugars, total	g	1.25	1.62
Minerals			
Calcium, Ca	mg	72	94
Iron, Fe	mg	0.9	1.17
Magnesium, Mg	mg	18	23
Phosphorus, P	mg	28	36
Potassium, K	mg	228	296
Sodium, Na	mg	23	30
Zinc, Zn	mg	0.24	0.31
Vitamins			

Vitamin C, total ascorbic acid	mg	41	53.3
Thiamin	mg	0.053	0.069
Riboflavin	mg	0.07	0.091
Niacin	mg	0.5	0.65
Vitamin B-6	mg	0.138	0.179
Folate, DFE	µg	13	17
Vitamin B-12	µg	0	0
Vitamin A, RAE	µg	681	885
Vitamin A, IU	IU	13621	17707
Vitamin E (alpha-tocopherol)	mg	0.85	1.1
Vitamin D (D2 + D3)	µg	0	0
Vitamin D	IU	0	0
Vitamin K (phylloquinone)	µg	817	1062.1
Lipids			
Fatty acids, total saturated	g	0.052	0.068
Fatty acids, total monounsaturated	g	0.03	0.039
Fatty acids, total polyunsaturated	g	0.193	0.251
Cholesterol	mg	0	0
Other			
Caffeine	mg	0	0

Source: USDA Nutrient Database

Chopped kale leaves are cooked with salt and water. Chopped leaves are taken in a pan and then water is added just to cover the leaves. Then a pinch of salt is also added. Leaves are cooked on a low flame for about 5 minutes until it is wilted and then drained it before consumption.

Nutrition in Cooked Kale (Boiled with salt and Drained)

Nutrient	Unit	Value per100g	1.0"cup, chopped"130.0g
Proximates			
Water	g	91.2	118.56
Energy	kcal	28	36
Protein	g	1.9	2.47
Total lipid (fat)	g	0.4	0.52

Carbohydrate, by difference	g	5.63	7.32
Fiber, total dietary	g	2	2.6
Sugars, total	g	1.25	1.62
Minerals			
Calcium, Ca	mg	72	94
Iron, Fe	mg	0.9	1.17
Magnesium, Mg	mg	18	23
Phosphorus, P	mg	28	36
Potassium, K	mg	228	296
Sodium, Na	mg	259	337
Zinc, Zn	mg	0.24	0.31
Vitamins			
Vitamin C, total ascorbic acid	mg	41	53.3
Thiamin	mg	0.053	0.069
Riboflavin	mg	0.07	0.091
Niacin	mg	0.5	0.65
Vitamin B-6	mg	0.138	0.179
Folate, DFE	µg	13	17
Vitamin B-12	µg	0	0
Vitamin A, RAE	µg	681	885
Vitamin A, IU	IU	13621	17707
Vitamin E (alpha-tocopherol)	mg	0.85	1.1
Vitamin D (D2 + D3)	µg	0	0
Vitamin D	IU	0	0
Lipids			
Fatty acids, total saturated	g	0.052	0.068
Fatty acids, total monounsaturated	g	0.03	0.039
Fatty acids, total polyunsaturated	g	0.193	0.251
Cholesterol	mg	0	0
Other			
Caffeine	mg	0	0

Source: USDA Nutrient Database

Nutrition in Frozen, Cooked Kale (Boiled without salt and Drained)

Nutrient	Unit	Value per 100g	1.0"cup, chopped"130.0g	0.5"cup, chopped or diced"65.0g
Proximates				
Water	g	90.5	117.65	58.82
Energy	kcal	30	39	20
Protein	g	2.84	3.69	1.85
Total lipid (fat)	g	0.49	0.64	0.32
Carbohydrate, by difference	g	5.23	6.8	3.4
Fiber, total dietary	g	2	2.6	1.3
Sugars, total	g	1.34	1.74	0.87
Minerals				
Calcium, Ca	mg	138	179	90
Iron, Fe	mg	0.94	1.22	0.61
Magnesium, Mg	mg	18	23	12
Phosphorus, P	mg	28	36	18
Potassium, K	mg	321	417	209
Sodium, Na	mg	15	20	10
Zinc, Zn	mg	0.18	0.23	0.12
Vitamins				
Vitamin C, total ascorbic acid	mg	25.2	32.8	16.4
Thiamin	mg	0.043	0.056	0.028
Riboflavin	mg	0.114	0.148	0.074
Niacin	mg	0.672	0.874	0.437
Vitamin B-6	mg	0.086	0.112	0.056
Folate, DFE	µg	14	18	9
Vitamin B-12	µg	0	0	0
Vitamin A, RAE	µg	735	956	478
Vitamin A, IU	IU	14704	19115	9558
Vitamin E (alpha-tocopherol)	mg	0.92	1.2	0.6
Vitamin D (D2 + D3)	µg	0	0	0
Vitamin D	IU	0	0	0

Vitamin K (phylloquinone)	Âμ g	882	1146.6	573.3
Lipids				
Fatty acids, total saturated	g	0.063	0.082	0.041
Fatty acids, total monounsaturated	g	0.036	0.047	0.023
Fatty acids, total polyunsaturated	g	0.235	0.306	0.153
Cholesterol	mg	0	0	0
Other				
Caffeine	mg	0	0	0

Source: USDA Nutrient Database

Nutrition in Frozen, Cooked Kale (Boiled with salt and Drained)

Nutrient	Unit	Value per100g	1.0"cup, chopped"130.0g
Proximates			
Water	g	90.5	117.65
Energy	kcal	30	39
Protein	g	2.84	3.69
Total lipid (fat)	g	0.49	0.64
Carbohydrate, by difference	g	5.23	6.8
Fiber, total dietary	g	2	2.6
Sugars, total	g	1.34	1.74
Minerals			
Calcium, Ca	mg	138	179
Iron, Fe	mg	0.94	1.22
Magnesium, Mg	mg	18	23
Phosphorus, P	mg	28	36
Potassium, K	mg	321	417
Sodium, Na	mg	251	326
Zinc, Zn	mg	0.18	0.23
Vitamins			
Vitamin C, total ascorbic acid	mg	25.2	32.8
Thiamin	mg	0.043	0.056
Riboflavin	mg	0.114	0.148

Niacin	mg	0.672	0.874
Vitamin B-6	mg	0.086	0.112
Folate, DFE	µg	14	18
Vitamin B-12	µg	0	0
Vitamin A, RAE	µg	735	956
Vitamin A, IU	IU	14704	19115
Vitamin E (alpha-tocopherol)	mg	0.92	1.2
Vitamin D (D2 + D3)	µg	0	0
Vitamin D	IU	0	0
Vitamin K (phylloquinone)	µg	882	1146.6
Lipids			
Fatty acids, total saturated	g	0.063	0.082
Fatty acids, total monounsaturated	g	0.036	0.047
Fatty acids, total polyunsaturated	g	0.235	0.306
Cholesterol	mg	0	0
Other			
Caffeine	mg	0	0

Source: USDA Nutrient Database

Scotch Kale

It is a curly-leaf variety of kale.

Nutrition in Raw (Fresh) Scotch Kale

Nutrient	Unit	Value per100g	1.0" cup, chopped" 67.0g
Water	g	87	58.29
Energy	kcal	42	28
Protein	g	2.8	1.88
Total lipid (fat)	g	0.6	0.4
Carbohydrate, by difference	g	8.32	5.57
Fiber, total dietary	g	1.7	1.1
Calcium, Ca	mg	205	137
Iron, Fe	mg	3	2.01
Magnesium, Mg	mg	88	59
Phosphorus, P	mg	62	42
Potassium, K	mg	450	302

Sodium, Na	mg	70	47
Zinc, Zn	mg	0.37	0.25
Vitamin C, total ascorbic acid	mg	130	87.1
Thiamin	mg	0.07	0.047
Riboflavin	mg	0.06	0.04
Niacin	mg	1.3	0.871
Vitamin B-6	mg	0.227	0.152
Folate, DFE	µg	28	19
Vitamin B-12	µg	0	0
Vitamin A, RAE	µg	155	104
Vitamin A, IU	IU	3100	2077
Vitamin D (D2 + D3)	µg	0	0
Vitamin D	IU	0	0
Fatty acids, total saturated	g	0.078	0.052
Fatty acids, total monounsaturated	g	0.045	0.03
Fatty acids, total polyunsaturated	g	0.289	0.194
Cholesterol	mg	0	0

Nutrition in Cooked Scotch Kale (Boiled without salt and Drained)

Nutrient	Unit	Value per100g	1.0"cup, chopped"130.0g
Water	g	91.2	118.56
Energy	kcal	28	36
Protein	g	1.9	2.47
Total lipid (fat)	g	0.41	0.53
Carbohydrate, by difference	g	5.63	7.32
Fiber, total dietary	g	1.2	1.6
Calcium, Ca	mg	132	172
Iron, Fe	mg	1.93	2.51
Magnesium, Mg	mg	57	74
Phosphorus, P	mg	38	49
Potassium, K	mg	274	356
Sodium, Na	mg	45	58
Zinc, Zn	mg	0.24	0.31
Vitamin C, total ascorbic acid	mg	52.8	68.6

Nutrient	Unit	Value	
Thiamin	mg	0.04	0.052
Riboflavin	mg	0.039	0.051
Niacin	mg	0.792	1.03
Vitamin B-6	mg	0.139	0.181
Folate, DFE	µg	13	17
Vitamin B-12	µg	0	0
Vitamin A, RAE	µg	100	130
Vitamin A, IU	IU	1994	2592
Vitamin D (D2 + D3)	µg	0	0
Vitamin D	IU	0	0
Fatty acids, total saturated	g	0.053	0.069
Fatty acids, total monounsaturated	g	0.03	0.039
Fatty acids, total polyunsaturated	g	0.196	0.255
Cholesterol	mg	0	0

Source: USDA Nutrient Database

Nutrition in Cooked Scotch Kale (Boiled with salt and Drained)

Nutrient	Unit	Value per100g	1.0"cup, chopped"130.0g
Water	g	91.2	118.56
Energy	kcal	28	36
Protein	g	1.9	2.47
Total lipid (fat)	g	0.41	0.53
Carbohydrate, by difference	g	5.62	7.31
Calcium, Ca	mg	132	172
Iron, Fe	mg	1.93	2.51
Magnesium, Mg	mg	57	74
Phosphorus, P	mg	38	49
Potassium, K	mg	274	356
Sodium, Na	mg	281	365
Zinc, Zn	mg	0.24	0.31
Vitamin C, total ascorbic acid	mg	52.8	68.6
Thiamin	mg	0.04	0.052
Riboflavin	mg	0.039	0.051
Niacin	mg	0.792	1.03

Vitamin B-6	mg	0.139	0.181
Folate, DFE	Âµg	13	17
Vitamin B-12	Âµg	0	0
Vitamin A, RAE	Âµg	100	130
Vitamin A, IU	IU	1994	2592
Vitamin D (D2 + D3)	Âµg	0	0
Vitamin D	IU	0	0
Fatty acids, total saturated	g	0.053	0.069
Fatty acids, total monounsaturated	g	0.03	0.039
Fatty acids, total polyunsaturated	g	0.196	0.255
Cholesterol	mg	0	0

Source: USDA Nutrient Database

Malabar Spinach or Indian Spinach

There are green-stemmed (Green Malabar) and red-stemmed (Red Malabar) varieties of Malabar spinach. Botanical name of green Malabar spinach is *Basella alba* and that of red Malabar spinach is *Basella rubra*. This plant belongs to family Basellaceae. It is a fast-growing herbaceous perennial plant and is edible. The leaves and tender shoots of the plant are used as a leafy vegetable. Even though it is a perennial plant it is grown as an annual or biennial for food purposes.

Malabar spinach is propagated via seeds or stem cuttings. It may be grown in open garden spaces where shade is available or as pot herbs. It may take 2-3 months for a seedling to reach harvest maturity. In case of stem cuttings, harvest maturity is reached within one to two months.

Malabar spinach is found growing abundantly in tropical continents such as Asia and Africa. It is believed to be originated in the tropical regions of Malabar Coast of India and Sri Lanka.

Other names of this plant are vine spinach, red vine spinach, creeping spinach, climbing spinach; buffalo spinach, Ceylon spinach, Surinam spinach, Chinese spinach, Vietnamese spinach, Malabar nightshade, Malabar green, and broad bologi. It is believed to be a native of the Indian Subcontinent and South East Asia.

Leaves are glossy, dark green, thick, succulent, and heart-shaped with a flavour. Leaves have a mucilaginous texture and rich in dietary fiber. Hence leaves may be used to thicken the consistency of soups. Malabar spinach may be cooked as stir-fries or as a main vegetable dish or as an additional ingredient in other vegetable preparations or as an ingredient in meat and fish preparations.

Nutrition in Raw Malabar Spinach

Nutrient	Unit	Value per100g
Water	g	93.1
Energy	kcal	19
Protein	g	1.8
Total lipid (fat)	g	0.3
Carbohydrate, by difference	g	3.4
Calcium, Ca	mg	109
Iron, Fe	mg	1.2
Magnesium, Mg	mg	65
Phosphorus, P	mg	52
Potassium, K	mg	510
Sodium, Na	mg	24
Zinc, Zn	mg	0.43
Vitamin C, total ascorbic acid	mg	102
Thiamin	mg	0.05
Riboflavin	mg	0.155
Niacin	mg	0.5
Vitamin B-6	mg	0.24
Folate, DFE	µg	140
Vitamin B-12	µg	0
Vitamin A, RAE	µg	400
Vitamin A, IU	IU	8000
Vitamin D (D2 + D3)	µg	0
Vitamin D	IU	0
Cholesterol	mg	0

Source: USDA Nutrient Database

Nutrition in Cooked Malabar Spinach

Nutrient	Unit	Value per100g	1.0"cup"44.0g	1.0"bunch"17.0g
Water	g	92.5	40.7	15.72
Energy	kcal	23	10	4
Protein	g	2.98	1.31	0.51
Total lipid (fat)	g	0.78	0.34	0.13
Carbohydrate, by difference	g	2.71	1.19	0.46
Fiber, total dietary	g	2.1	0.9	0.4
Calcium, Ca	mg	124	55	21
Iron, Fe	mg	1.48	0.65	0.25
Magnesium, Mg	mg	48	21	8
Phosphorus, P	mg	36	16	6
Potassium, K	mg	256	113	44
Sodium, Na	mg	55	24	9
Zinc, Zn	mg	0.3	0.13	0.05
Vitamin C, total ascorbic acid	mg	5.9	2.6	1
Thiamin	mg	0.106	0.047	0.018
Riboflavin	mg	0.129	0.057	0.022
Niacin	mg	0.787	0.346	0.134
Vitamin B-6	mg	0.086	0.038	0.015
Folate, DFE	Âµg	114	50	19
Vitamin B-12	Âµg	0	0	0
Vitamin A, RAE	Âµg	58	26	10
Vitamin A, IU	IU	1158	510	197
Vitamin D (D2 + D3)	Âµg	0	0	0
Vitamin D	IU	0	0	0
Cholesterol	mg	0	0	0

Source: USDA Nutrient Database

62

Mustard Spinach

Scientific name of Mustard spinach is *Brassica rapa* and it belongs to the family Brassicaceae. Mustard spinach is considered as a highly nutritious leafy vegetable. Detailed nutritional information per 100 grams of edible portion is given below.

Nutrition in Raw Mustard Spinach (tender green mustard)

Nutrient	Unit	Value per100g	1.0"cup, chopped"150.0g
Water	g	92.2	138.3
Energy	kcal	22	33
Protein	g	2.2	3.3
Total lipid (fat)	g	0.3	0.45
Carbohydrate, by difference	g	3.9	5.85
Fiber, total dietary	g	2.8	4.2
Calcium, Ca	mg	210	315
Iron, Fe	mg	1.5	2.25
Magnesium, Mg	mg	11	16
Phosphorus, P	mg	28	42
Potassium, K	mg	449	674
Sodium, Na	mg	21	32
Zinc, Zn	mg	0.17	0.26
Vitamin C, total ascorbic acid	mg	130	195
Thiamin	mg	0.068	0.102
Riboflavin	mg	0.093	0.139
Niacin	mg	0.678	1.017
Vitamin B-6	mg	0.153	0.229
Folate, DFE	µg	159	238
Vitamin B-12	µg	0	0
Vitamin A, RAE	µg	495	742
Vitamin A, IU	IU	9900	14850

Vitamin D (D2 + D3)	µg	0	0
Vitamin D	IU	0	0
Fatty acids, total saturated	g	0.015	0.022
Fatty acids, total monounsaturated	g	0.138	0.207
Fatty acids, total polyunsaturated	g	0.057	0.086
Cholesterol	mg	0	0

Source: USDA Nutrient Database

Nutrition in Cooked (by Boiling without Salt) Mustard Spinach

Nutrient	Unit	Value per100g	1.0"cup, chopped"180.0g
Water	g	94.5	170.1
Energy	kcal	16	29
Protein	g	1.7	3.06
Total lipid (fat)	g	0.2	0.36
Carbohydrate, by difference	g	2.8	5.04
Fiber, total dietary	g	2	3.6
Calcium, Ca	mg	158	284
Iron, Fe	mg	0.8	1.44
Magnesium, Mg	mg	7	13
Phosphorus, P	mg	18	32
Potassium, K	mg	285	513
Sodium, Na	mg	14	25
Zinc, Zn	mg	0.11	0.2
Vitamin C, total ascorbic acid	mg	65	117
Thiamin	mg	0.041	0.074
Riboflavin	mg	0.062	0.112
Niacin	mg	0.43	0.774
Vitamin B-6	mg	0.097	0.175
Folate, DFE	µg	73	131
Vitamin B-12	µg	0	0
Vitamin A, RAE	µg	410	738
Vitamin A, IU	IU	8200	14760
Cholesterol	mg	0	0

Source: USDA Nutrient Database

Mustard Leaves or Mustard Greens

Scientific name of mustard greens is *Brassica juncea* and it belongs to the family Brassicaceae. Even though leaves, stems and seeds of the mustard plant are edible, here focus is on tender green mustard leaves.

Mustard leaves are dark green in colour and with a strong flavour. Greens are popularly used for cooking a delicious leafy vegetable dish called '*sarson da saag*' in many Asian countries. This vegetable dish is consumed along with *chapati* (wheat bread) or steamed rice.

Mustard leaves may be cooked along with other vegetable greens such as dandelion greens, mustard spinach etc in order to reduce its strong flavour.

Nutrition in Raw Mustard Greens

Nutrient	Unit	Value per100g	1.0"cup, chopped"56.0g
Water	g	90.7	50.79
Energy	kcal	27	15
Protein	g	2.86	1.6
Total lipid (fat)	g	0.42	0.24
Carbohydrate, by difference	g	4.67	2.62
Fiber, total dietary	g	3.2	1.8
Sugars, total	g	1.32	0.74
Minerals			
Calcium, Ca	mg	115	64
Iron, Fe	mg	1.64	0.92
Magnesium, Mg	mg	32	18
Phosphorus, P	mg	58	32
Potassium, K	mg	384	215
Sodium, Na	mg	20	11
Zinc, Zn	mg	0.25	0.14

Vitamins			
Vitamin C, total ascorbic acid	mg	70	39.2
Thiamin	mg	0.08	0.045
Riboflavin	mg	0.11	0.062
Niacin	mg	0.8	0.448
Vitamin B-6	mg	0.18	0.101
Folate, DFE	µg	12	7
Vitamin B-12	µg	0	0
Vitamin A, RAE	µg	151	85
Vitamin A, IU	IU	3024	1693
Vitamin E (alpha-tocopherol)	mg	2.01	1.13
Vitamin D (D2 + D3)	µg	0	0
Vitamin D	IU	0	0
Vitamin K (phylloquinone)	µg	257.5	144.2
Lipids			
Fatty acids, total saturated	g	0.01	0.006
Fatty acids, total monounsaturated	g	0.092	0.052
Fatty acids, total polyunsaturated	g	0.038	0.021
Cholesterol	mg	0	0
Other			
Caffeine	mg	0	0

Source: USDA Nutrient Database

66

Nutrition in Cooked Mustard Greens (boiled, drained, without salt)

Nutrient	Unit	Value per100g	1.0"cup, chopped"140.0g
Water	g	91.78	128.49
Energy	kcal	26	36
Protein	g	2.56	3.58
Total lipid (fat)	g	0.47	0.66
Carbohydrate, by difference	g	4.51	6.31
Fiber, total dietary	g	2	2.8
Sugars, total	g	1.41	1.97
Calcium, Ca	mg	118	165
Iron, Fe	mg	0.87	1.22
Magnesium, Mg	mg	13	18
Phosphorus, P	mg	42	59
Potassium, K	mg	162	227
Sodium, Na	mg	9	13
Zinc, Zn	mg	0.22	0.31
Vitamin C, total ascorbic acid	mg	25.3	35.4
Thiamin	mg	0.041	0.057
Riboflavin	mg	0.063	0.088
Niacin	mg	0.433	0.606
Vitamin B-6	mg	0.098	0.137
Folate, DFE	µg	9	13
Vitamin B-12	µg	0	0
Vitamin A, RAE	µg	618	865
Vitamin A, IU	IU	12370	17318
Vitamin E (alpha-tocopherol)	mg	1.78	2.49
Vitamin D (D2 + D3)	µg	0	0
Vitamin D	IU	0	0
Vitamin K (phylloquinone)	µg	592.7	829.8
Fatty acids, total saturated	g	0.012	0.017
Fatty acids, total monounsaturated	g	0.11	0.154
Fatty acids, total polyunsaturated	g	0.046	0.064

Source: USDA Nutrient Database

Nutrition in Frozen Unprepared Mustard Greens

Nutrient	Unit	Value per100g	1.0"cup, chopped"146.0g	1.0"package (10 oz)"284.0g
Water	g	93.21	136.09	264.72
Energy	kcal	20	29	57
Protein	g	2.49	3.64	7.07
Total lipid (fat)	g	0.27	0.39	0.77
Carbohydrate, by difference	g	3.41	4.98	9.68
Fiber, total dietary	g	3.3	4.8	9.4
Calcium, Ca	mg	116	169	329
Iron, Fe	mg	1.29	1.88	3.66
Magnesium, Mg	mg	15	22	43
Phosphorus, P	mg	30	44	85
Potassium, K	mg	170	248	483
Sodium, Na	mg	29	42	82
Zinc, Zn	mg	0.23	0.34	0.65
Vitamin C, total ascorbic acid	mg	25.3	36.9	71.9
Thiamin	mg	0.048	0.07	0.136
Riboflavin	mg	0.061	0.089	0.173
Niacin	mg	0.314	0.458	0.892
Vitamin B-6	mg	0.131	0.191	0.372
Folate, DFE	µg	138	201	392
Vitamin B-12	µg	0	0	0
Vitamin A, RAE	µg	258	377	733
Vitamin A, IU	IU	5155	7526	14640
Vitamin D (D2 + D3)	µg	0	0	0
Vitamin D	IU	0	0	0
Fatty acids, total saturated	g	0.014	0.02	0.04
Fatty acids, total monounsaturated	g	0.124	0.181	0.352
Fatty acids, total polyunsaturated	g	0.051	0.074	0.145

Source: USDA Nutrient Database

Nutrition in Frozen Mustard Greens (cooked, boiled, drained, without salt

Nutrient	Unit	Value per100g	1.0"cup, chopped"150.0g	1.0"package (10 oz) yields"212.0g
Water	g	93.8	140.7	198.86
Energy	kcal	19	28	40
Protein	g	2.27	3.4	4.81
Total lipid (fat)	g	0.25	0.38	0.53
Carbohydrate, by difference	g	3.11	4.66	6.59
Fiber, total dietary	g	2.8	4.2	5.9
Sugars, total	g	0.32	0.48	0.68
Calcium, Ca	mg	101	152	214
Iron, Fe	mg	1.12	1.68	2.37
Magnesium, Mg	mg	13	20	28
Phosphorus, P	mg	24	36	51
Potassium, K	mg	139	208	295
Sodium, Na	mg	25	38	53
Zinc, Zn	mg	0.2	0.3	0.42
Vitamin C, total ascorbic acid	mg	13.8	20.7	29.3
Thiamin	mg	0.04	0.06	0.085
Riboflavin	mg	0.053	0.08	0.112
Niacin	mg	0.258	0.387	0.547
Vitamin B-6	mg	0.108	0.162	0.229
Folate, DFE	Âµg	70	105	148
Vitamin A, RAE	Âµg	354	531	750
Vitamin A, IU	IU	7076	10614	15001
Vitamin E (alpha-tocopherol)	mg	1.35	2.02	2.86
Vitamin K (phylloquinone)	Âµg	335.1	502.6	710.4
Fatty acids, total saturated	g	0.013	0.02	0.028
Fatty acids, total monounsaturated	g	0.113	0.169	0.24
Fatty acids, total polyunsaturated	g	0.047	0.07	0.1

Source: USDA Nutrient Database

New Zealand Spinach

Scientific name of New Zealand spinach is Tetragonia tetragonioides (syn. T. expansa) and it belongs to the family Aizoaceae. It is a trailing annual plant, leaves of which are used as a vegetable. Leaves are thick, triangular-shaped, bright green in colour and with a lettuce-like flavour.

New Zealand spinach is also known as tetragonia, ice plant, everbearing spinach, everlasting spinach, perpetual spinach, Della Nuova Zelanda

Warrigal greens, Warrigal cabbage, sea spinach, Botany Bay spinach, tetragon and Cook's cabbage. It is native to New Zealand, Australia, Japan, Chile and Argentina.

Raw leaves are not suitable for consumption because of the presence of oxalates in them which may be allergic to some people. Blanching of leaves is done to remove oxalates just before cooking the leaves. Blanching is a process where freshly harvested leaves are immersed in hot water for a minute and then these leaves are rinsed with cold water.

New Zealand spinach is cooked as a major vegetable dish or may be pickled. Blanched leaves may be used as an ingredient in salads. It may also be used in soups and stews. It may be added as an ingredient in pastas and omelettes.

It is low in calories, proteins, and carbohydrates and fat, but high in nutrients. It is an excellent source of vitamin A, with 4,400 international units (IU) per 100 gram. Other notable vitamins include 30 mg of vitamin C per 100 gram of edible portion.

It is rich in minerals such as 130 milligrams each of sodium and potassium in 100 grams of edible portion and 58 milligrams of calcium, 39 milligrams of magnesium and 28 milligrams of phosphorous in 100 grams of edible portion.

Nutritional Information for Raw New Zealand Spinach

Nutrient	Unit	Value per100g	1.0"cup, chopped"56.0g
Water	g	94	52.64
Energy	kcal	14	8
Protein	g	1.5	0.84
Total lipid (fat)	g	0.2	0.11
Carbohydrate, by difference	g	2.5	1.4
Fiber, total dietary	g	1.5	0.8
Sugars, total	g	0.29	0.16
Calcium, Ca	mg	58	32
Iron, Fe	mg	0.8	0.45
Magnesium, Mg	mg	39	22
Phosphorus, P	mg	28	16
Potassium, K	mg	130	73
Sodium, Na	mg	130	73
Zinc, Zn	mg	0.38	0.21
Vitamin C, total ascorbic acid	mg	30	16.8
Thiamin	mg	0.04	0.022
Riboflavin	mg	0.13	0.073
Niacin	mg	0.5	0.28
Vitamin B-6	mg	0.304	0.17
Folate, DFE	Âµg	15	8
Vitamin B-12	Âµg	0	0
Vitamin A, IU	IU	4400	2464
Vitamin E (alpha-tocopherol)	mg	1.42	0.8
Vitamin D (D2 + D3)	Âµg	0	0
Vitamin D	IU	0	0
Vitamin K (phylloquinone)	Âµg	337	188.7
Fatty acids, total saturated	g	0.032	0.018
Fatty acids, total monounsaturated	g	0.005	0.003
Fatty acids, total polyunsaturated	g	0.084	0.047
Cholesterol	mg	0	0
Caffeine	mg	0	0

Source: USDA Nutrient Database

Nutrition in Cooked New Zealand Spinach (boiled, drained, without salt)

Nutrient	Unit	Value per100g	1.0"cup, chopped"180.0g
Water	g	94.8	170.64
Energy	kcal	12	22
Protein	g	1.3	2.34
Total lipid (fat)	g	0.17	0.31
Carbohydrate, by difference	g	2.13	3.83
Fiber, total dietary	g	1.4	2.5
Sugars, total	g	0.25	0.45
Calcium, Ca	mg	48	86
Iron, Fe	mg	0.66	1.19
Magnesium, Mg	mg	32	58
Phosphorus, P	mg	22	40
Potassium, K	mg	102	184
Sodium, Na	mg	107	193
Zinc, Zn	mg	0.31	0.56
Vitamin C, total ascorbic acid	mg	16	28.8
Thiamin	mg	0.03	0.054
Riboflavin	mg	0.107	0.193
Niacin	mg	0.39	0.702
Vitamin B-6	mg	0.237	0.427
Folate, DFE	µg	8	14
Vitamin B-12	µg	0	0
Vitamin A, IU	IU	3622	6520
Vitamin E (alpha-tocopherol)	mg	1.23	2.21
Vitamin D (D2 + D3)	µg	0	0
Vitamin D	IU	0	0
Vitamin K (phylloquinone)	µg	292	525.6
Fatty acids, total saturated	g	0.027	0.049
Fatty acids, total monounsaturated	g	0.005	0.009
Fatty acids, total polyunsaturated	g	0.071	0.128

Source: USDA Nutrient Database

Pumpkin Leaves

Pumpkin leaves are harvested along with the tips that attach to the vine. That is, leaves and tips are harvested together and both are edible. Pumpkin leaves are rich in iron, protein, calcium, vitamin A and vitamin C, and are used for preparing salads, soups, and stir fries.

Nutrition in Raw Pumpkin Leaves

Nutrient	Unit	Value per100g	1.0"cup"39.0g
Water	g	92.88	36.22
Energy	kcal	19	7
Protein	g	3.15	1.23
Total lipid (fat)	g	0.4	0.16
Carbohydrate, by difference	g	2.33	0.91
Calcium, Ca	mg	39	15
Iron, Fe	mg	2.22	0.87
Magnesium, Mg	mg	38	15
Phosphorus, P	mg	104	41
Potassium, K	mg	436	170
Sodium, Na	mg	11	4
Zinc, Zn	mg	0.2	0.08
Vitamin C, total ascorbic acid	mg	11	4.3
Thiamin	mg	0.094	0.037
Riboflavin	mg	0.128	0.05
Niacin	mg	0.92	0.359
Vitamin B-6	mg	0.207	0.081
Folate, DFE	Âµg	36	14
Vitamin A, RAE	Âµg	97	38
Vitamin A, IU	IU	1942	757
Fatty acids, total saturated	g	0.207	0.081
Fatty acids, total monounsaturated	g	0.052	0.02
Fatty acids, total polyunsaturated	g	0.022	0.009

Source: USDA Nutrient Database

Nutrition in Cooked Pumpkin Leaves (boiled, drained, without salt)

Nutrient	Unit	Value per100g	1.0"cup"71.0g
Water	g	92.51	65.68
Energy	kcal	21	15
Protein	g	2.72	1.93
Total lipid (fat)	g	0.22	0.16
Carbohydrate, by difference	g	3.39	2.41
Fiber, total dietary	g	2.7	1.9
Sugars, total	g	0.69	0.49
Calcium, Ca	mg	43	31
Iron, Fe	mg	3.2	2.27
Magnesium, Mg	mg	38	27
Phosphorus, P	mg	79	56
Potassium, K	mg	438	311
Sodium, Na	mg	8	6
Zinc, Zn	mg	0.2	0.14
Vitamin C, total ascorbic acid	mg	1	0.7
Thiamin	mg	0.068	0.048
Riboflavin	mg	0.136	0.097
Niacin	mg	0.85	0.604
Vitamin B-6	mg	0.196	0.139
Folate, DFE	Åμg	25	18
Vitamin B-12	Åμg	0	0
Vitamin A, RAE	Åμg	80	57
Vitamin A, IU	IU	1600	1136
Vitamin E (alpha-tocopherol)	mg	0.96	0.68
Vitamin K (phylloquinone)	Åμg	108	76.7
Fatty acids, total saturated	g	0.114	0.081
Fatty acids, total monounsaturated	g	0.029	0.021
Fatty acids, total polyunsaturated	g	0.012	0.009

Source: USDA Nutrient Database

Nutrition in Cooked Pumpkin Leaves (boiled, drained, with salt)

Nutrient	Unit	Value per100g	1.0"cup"71.0g
Water	g	92.51	65.68
Energy	kcal	21	15
Protein	g	2.72	1.93
Total lipid (fat)	g	0.22	0.16
Carbohydrate, by difference	g	3.39	2.41
Fiber, total dietary	g	2.7	1.9
Sugars, total	g	0.69	0.49
Calcium, Ca	mg	43	31
Iron, Fe	mg	3.2	2.27
Magnesium, Mg	mg	38	27
Phosphorus, P	mg	79	56
Potassium, K	mg	438	311
Sodium, Na	mg	244	173
Zinc, Zn	mg	0.2	0.14
Vitamin C, total ascorbic acid	mg	1	0.7
Thiamin	mg	0.068	0.048
Riboflavin	mg	0.136	0.097
Niacin	mg	0.85	0.604
Vitamin B-6	mg	0.196	0.139
Folate, DFE	µg	25	18
Vitamin B-12	µg	0	0
Vitamin A, RAE	µg	80	57
Vitamin A, IU	IU	1600	1136
Vitamin E (alpha-tocopherol)	mg	0.96	0.68
Vitamin K (phylloquinone)	µg	108	76.7
Fatty acids, total saturated	g	0.114	0.081
Fatty acids, total monounsaturated	g	0.029	0.021
Fatty acids, total polyunsaturated	g	0.012	0.009
Cholesterol	mg	0	0
Caffeine	mg	0	0

Source: USDA Nutrient Database

Purslane or Portulaca

Scientific name of purslane is *Portulaca oleracea* and it belongs to the family *Portulacaceae*. It is believed to be originated in the Indian subcontinent. It is an annual herbaceous plant with succulent leaves and stems.

Nutrition in Raw Purslane (Portulaca)

Nutrient	Unit	1Value per100g	1.0"cup"43.0g	1.0"plant"3.0g
Water	g	92.86	39.93	2.79
Energy	kcal	20	9	1
Protein	g	2.03	0.87	0.06
Total lipid (fat)	g	0.36	0.15	0.01
Carbohydrate, by difference	g	3.39	1.46	0.1
Calcium, Ca	mg	65	28	2
Iron, Fe	mg	1.99	0.86	0.06
Magnesium, Mg	mg	68	29	2
Phosphorus, P	mg	44	19	1
Potassium, K	mg	494	212	15
Sodium, Na	mg	45	19	1
Zinc, Zn	mg	0.17	0.07	0.01
Vitamin C, total ascorbic acid	mg	21	9	0.6
Thiamin	mg	0.047	0.02	0.001
Riboflavin	mg	0.112	0.048	0.003
Niacin	mg	0.48	0.206	0.014
Vitamin B-6	mg	0.073	0.031	0.002
Folate, DFE	Âµg	12	5	0
Vitamin A, IU	IU	1320	568	40
Cholesterol	mg	0	0	0

Source: USDA Nutrient Database

76

Nutrition in Cooked Purslane (boiled, drained, without salt)

Nutrient	Unit	Value per100g	1.0"cup"115.0 g	1.0"squash"431.0 g
Water	g	93.52	107.55	403.07
Energy	kcal	18	21	78
Protein	g	1.49	1.71	6.42
Total lipid (fat)	g	0.19	0.22	0.82
Carbohydrate, by difference	g	3.55	4.08	15.3
Calcium, Ca	mg	78	90	336
Iron, Fe	mg	0.77	0.89	3.32
Magnesium, Mg	mg	67	77	289
Phosphorus, P	mg	37	43	159
Potassium, K	mg	488	561	2103
Sodium, Na	mg	44	51	190
Zinc, Zn	mg	0.17	0.2	0.73
Vitamin C, total ascorbic acid	mg	10.5	12.1	45.3
Thiamin	mg	0.031	0.036	0.134
Riboflavin	mg	0.09	0.104	0.388
Niacin	mg	0.46	0.529	1.983
Vitamin B-6	mg	0.07	0.08	0.302
Folate, DFE	µg	9	10	39
Vitamin B-12	µg	0	0	0
Vitamin A, RAE	µg	93	107	401
Vitamin A, IU	IU	1852	2130	7982

Source: USDA Nutrient Database

Swisschard

Scientific name of Swiss chard is *Beta vulgaris* var. *cicla* and it belongs to the family Chenopodiaceae, the beet leaf family. Swiss chard, a vegetable of temperate climate, is believed to be originated in Mediterranean region.

It is mainly grown for its edible leaves which are used as a leafy vegetable. Leaves look like spinach leaves but larger and with white veins. Tender, young leaves are used as a salad vegetable while large mature leaves and stalks are used for cooking as a vegetable.

Nutrition in Raw Swisschard

Nutrient	Unit	Value per100g	1.0"cup"36.0 g	1.0"leaf"48.0 g
Water	g	92.66	33.36	44.48
Energy	kcal	19	7	9
Protein	g	1.8	0.65	0.86
Total lipid (fat)	g	0.2	0.07	0.1
Carbohydrate, by difference	g	3.74	1.35	1.8
Fiber, total dietary	g	1.6	0.6	0.8
Sugars, total	g	1.1	0.4	0.53
Calcium, Ca	mg	51	18	24
Iron, Fe	mg	1.8	0.65	0.86
Magnesium, Mg	mg	81	29	39
Phosphorus, P	mg	46	17	22
Potassium, K	mg	379	136	182
Sodium, Na	mg	213	77	102
Zinc, Zn	mg	0.36	0.13	0.17
Vitamin C, total ascorbic acid	mg	30	10.8	14.4
Thiamin	mg	0.04	0.014	0.019
Riboflavin	mg	0.09	0.032	0.043
Niacin	mg	0.4	0.144	0.192
Vitamin B-6	mg	0.099	0.036	0.048
Folate, DFE	Âµg	14	5	7
Vitamin A, RAE	Âµg	306	110	147
Vitamin A, IU	IU	6116	2202	2936
Vitamin E (alpha-tocopherol)	mg	1.89	0.68	0.91
Vitamin K (phylloquinone)	Âµg	830	298.8	398.4
Fatty acids, total saturated	g	0.03	0.011	0.014
Fatty acids, total monounsaturated	g	0.04	0.014	0.019
Fatty acids, total polyunsaturated	g	0.07	0.025	0.034

Source: USDA Nutrient Database

Nutrition in Cooked Swisschard (boiled, drained, without salt)

Nutrient	Unit	Value per100g	1.0"cup, chopped"175.0g
Water	g	92.65	162.14
Energy	kcal	20	35
Protein	g	1.88	3.29
Total lipid (fat)	g	0.08	0.14
Carbohydrate, by difference	g	4.13	7.23
Fiber, total dietary	g	2.1	3.7
Sugars, total	g	1.1	1.93
Calcium, Ca	mg	58	102
Iron, Fe	mg	2.26	3.95
Magnesium, Mg	mg	86	150
Phosphorus, P	mg	33	58
Potassium, K	mg	549	961
Sodium, Na	mg	179	313
Zinc, Zn	mg	0.33	0.58
Vitamin C, total ascorbic acid	mg	18	31.5
Thiamin	mg	0.034	0.06
Riboflavin	mg	0.086	0.15
Niacin	mg	0.36	0.63
Vitamin B-6	mg	0.085	0.149
Folate, DFE	µg	9	16
Vitamin B-12	µg	0	0
Vitamin A, RAE	µg	306	536
Vitamin A, IU	IU	6124	10717
Vitamin E (alpha-tocopherol)	mg	1.89	3.31
Vitamin K (phylloquinone)	µg	327.3	572.8
Fatty acids, total saturated	g	0.012	0.021
Fatty acids, total monounsaturated	g	0.016	0.028
Fatty acids, total polyunsaturated	g	0.028	0.049
Cholesterol	mg	0	0

Source: USDA Nutrient Database

Seakale

Scientific name of seakale is *Crambe maritime* and it belongs to cabbage family or mustard family i.e. *Brassicaceae (syn.* Cruciferae). In other words, seakale is a brassica vegetable or a cruciferous vegetable.

Brassica vegetables are biennial in their growing habit but for food purposes they are grown as annuals. Brassica vegetables believed to be originated in the region comprising of Western Europe, the Mediterranean region and the temperate regions of Asia.

Seakale is a hardy plant, leaves of which resemble to that of plants of cabbage family. Leaves are serrated and bluish green in colour. Young leaves and shoots of seakale are used as a leafy vegetable.

Raw leaves are not suitable for consumption. Generally, blanched leaves of seakale are used for cooking as a vegetable.

Just like other brassica vegetables, Seakale leaves are rich in dietary fiber, vitamins and minerals and low in fatty acids and cholesterol. It is rich in minerals like iodine, sulfur, Calcium, Potassium and Magnesium. Since seakale leaves are rich in Vitamin C, consumption of which is advised in cases of scurvy. Seakale leaves are also rich in Vitamin A and Carotenoids (carotene is a precursor of Vitamin A). Consumption of seakale leaves is also helps in alleviating health disorders such as osteoporosis, some heart disorders and dementia.

Health Benefits of Seakale and other Brassica Vegetables

Brassica vegetables are considered to be the richest source of plant-based antioxidants in a human diet. An antioxidant is a substance that inhibits oxidation, especially that of free radicals. Free radicals are chemically unstable molecular fragments or atoms that have a charge due to excess or deficient number of electrons and are directly responsible for cell degeneration and resultant ageing process in human beings. The immediate tendency of free radicals, as soon as they are formed, is to become stable by reacting with cellular components (for example: DNA) or cell membrane. The result is DNA damage, malignant tumour formation (cancer) and diabetes, cataract, heart diseases and other cell degenerative diseases. Some of the examples of free radicals are superoxide

81

anion, hydroxyl radical, transition metals such as iron and copper, nitric acid and ozone. Major sources of free radicals are normal oxidation process happening within the human body (i.e. released as a byproduct of cell metabolism), exposure to pollution (free radicals may be present in the air we breathe), exposure to sunlight and lifestyle factors such as alcohol consumption, wrong diet habits (free radicals may be present in the food we eat), stress, and smoking. Some of the examples of cell damage by free radicals are cataract (lens of the eyes become opaque), damage to cell's protective lipid layer (cell membrane), and heart diseases where free radicals trap LDL (low density lipoprotein) in blood artery walls and form coatings.

Antioxidants are present in the form of vitamins, minerals, enzymes and polyphenolic compounds. Major Antioxidant Vitamins are Vitamin C and Vitamin E. brassica vegetables such as broccoli, brussels sprouts, cauliflower, and kale are rich source of Vitamin C. This vitamin is water soluble, easily absorbed by the body hence a mighty scavenger of free radicals present in the bodily fluids including blood. Broccoli is rich in Vitamin E which is essential for the prevention of oxidation of lipids (fats). Major antioxidant minerals are Zinc and Selenium. Selenium is essential to form an active site of most antioxidant enzymes. Major antioxidant enzymes present in human body are Superoxide Dismutase (SOD), catalase (CAT) and Glutathione and glutathione peroxidise. All these three groups of antioxidant enzymes are working together to protect cells from free radical damage.

Polyphenolic compounds or polyphenols are a large group comprising of flavonoids, carotenoids, and anthocyanins. Flavonoids are chemical compounds plants produce to protect themselves from cell damage and it is a subgroup of polyphenolic antioxidants. It reduces cell inflammation, improves memory and concentration and increases body's immunity. Anthocyanins are a subgroup of flavonoids. In case of carotenoids, there are about 600 types of carotenoids known till date. Some of these are alpha carotene, beta carotene, lycopene, cryptoxanthin, zeaxanthin, and lutein. Beta carotene is the most studied carotenoids and is a precursor of Vitamin A. brassica vegetables such as broccoli, kale, and collard greens are rich source of beta carotene.

Sweet Potato Leaves

Botanical name of sweet potato is *Ipomoea batatas* and it belongs to the family Convolvulaceae. It is a trailing herbaceous plant which is perennial in its growth habit. Young, tender sweet potato leaves are used as a leafy vegetable. According to Food and Agriculture Organization, sweet potato leaves are a good source of vitamins A, C, and B2 (riboflavin), and lutein.

Nutrition in Raw Sweet Potato Leaves

Nutrient	Unit	Value per100g	1.0"cup, chopped"35.0g	1.0"leaf (12-1/4" long)"16.0g
Water	g	86.81	30.38	13.89
Energy	kcal	42	15	7
Protein	g	2.49	0.87	0.4
Total lipid (fat)	g	0.51	0.18	0.08
Carbohydrate, by difference	g	8.82	3.09	1.41
Fiber, total dietary	g	5.3	1.9	0.8
Calcium, Ca	mg	78	27	12
Iron, Fe	mg	0.97	0.34	0.16
Magnesium, Mg	mg	70	24	11
Phosphorus, P	mg	81	28	13
Potassium, K	mg	508	178	81
Sodium, Na	mg	6	2	1
Vitamin C, total ascorbic acid	mg	11	3.8	1.8
Thiamin	mg	0.156	0.055	0.025
Riboflavin	mg	0.345	0.121	0.055
Niacin	mg	1.13	0.395	0.181
Vitamin B-6	mg	0.19	0.066	0.03
Folate, DFE	µg	1	0	0
Vitamin A, RAE	µg	189	66	30
Vitamin A, IU	IU	3778	1322	604
Vitamin K (phylloquinone)	µg	302.2	105.8	48.4
Fatty acids, total saturated	g	0.111	0.039	0.018
Fatty acids, total monounsaturated	g	0.02	0.007	0.003
Fatty acids, total polyunsaturated	g	0.228	0.08	0.036

83

Nutrition in Cooked Sweet Potato Leaves (steamed, without salt)

Nutrient	Unit	Value per100g	1.0"cup"64.0g
Water	g	89.2	57.09
Energy	kcal	41	26
Protein	g	2.18	1.4
Total lipid (fat)	g	0.34	0.22
Carbohydrate, by difference	g	7.38	4.72
Fiber, total dietary	g	1.9	1.2
Sugars, total	g	5.48	3.51
Calcium, Ca	mg	33	21
Iron, Fe	mg	0.63	0.4
Magnesium, Mg	mg	48	31
Phosphorus, P	mg	40	26
Potassium, K	mg	312	200
Sodium, Na	mg	7	4
Zinc, Zn	mg	0.26	0.17
Vitamin C, total ascorbic acid	mg	1.5	1
Thiamin	mg	0.112	0.072
Riboflavin	mg	0.267	0.171
Niacin	mg	1.003	0.642
Vitamin B-6	mg	0.16	0.102
Folate, DFE	µg	49	31
Vitamin B-12	µg	0	0
Vitamin A, RAE	µg	147	94
Vitamin A, IU	IU	2939	1881
Vitamin E (alpha-tocopherol)	mg	0.96	0.61
Vitamin K (phylloquinone)	µg	108.6	69.5
Fatty acids, total saturated	g	0.065	0.042
Fatty acids, total monounsaturated	g	0.012	0.008
Fatty acids, total polyunsaturated	g	0.134	0.086
Cholesterol	mg	0	0

Source: USDA Nutrient Database

Nutrition in Cooked Sweet Potato Leaves (steamed, with salt)

Nutrient	Unit	Value per100g	1.0"cup"64.0g
Water	g	89.2	57.09
Energy	kcal	35	22
Protein	g	2.18	1.4
Total lipid (fat)	g	0.34	0.22
Carbohydrate, by difference	g	7.38	4.72
Fiber, total dietary	g	1.9	1.2
Sugars, total	g	5.48	3.51
Calcium, Ca	mg	33	21
Iron, Fe	mg	0.63	0.4
Magnesium, Mg	mg	48	31
Phosphorus, P	mg	40	26
Potassium, K	mg	312	200
Sodium, Na	mg	249	159
Zinc, Zn	mg	0.26	0.17
Vitamin C, total ascorbic acid	mg	1.5	1
Thiamin	mg	0.112	0.072
Riboflavin	mg	0.267	0.171
Niacin	mg	1.003	0.642
Vitamin B-6	mg	0.16	0.102
Folate, DFE	Âµg	49	31
Vitamin B-12	Âµg	0	0
Vitamin A, RAE	Âµg	147	94
Vitamin A, IU	IU	2939	1881
Vitamin E (alpha-tocopherol)	mg	0.96	0.61
Vitamin K (phylloquinone)	Âµg	108.6	69.5
Fatty acids, total saturated	g	0.065	0.042
Fatty acids, total monounsaturated	g	0.012	0.008
Fatty acids, total polyunsaturated	g	0.134	0.086
Cholesterol	mg	0	0

Source: USDA Nutrient Database

Winged Bean Leaves

Winged beans or winged pea is a tropical, herbaceous, perennial, leguminaceous climber (a plant with trailing stems). Scientific name of winged bean is *Psophocarpus tetragonolobus* and it belongs to the family leguminaceae. Even though winged bean is perennial in growth habit, it is grown as an annual climber for food purposes.

Winged bean is also known as Manila beans and Mauritius beans as it is found growing abundantly in these regions. It is also known as four-angled bean as each bean pod has four wings with distinctly marked corners or edges.

Winged bean leaves, shape of which varies from ovate to lanceolate, may be used as a nutritious leafy vegetable. Young, tender leaves are used as an ingredient in soups, stews, vegetable preparations etc. Chopped raw leaves may be used in salads. Cooking is almost similar to that of spinach.

Nutrition in Raw, Winged Bean Leaves

Nutrient	Unit	Value per 100g
Water	g	76.85
Energy	kcal	74
Protein	g	5.85
Total lipid (fat)	g	1.1
Carbohydrate, by difference	g	14.1
Calcium, Ca	mg	224
Iron, Fe	mg	4
Magnesium, Mg	mg	8
Phosphorus, P	mg	63
Potassium, K	mg	176
Sodium, Na	mg	9
Zinc, Zn	mg	1.28
Vitamin C, total ascorbic acid	mg	45
Thiamin	mg	0.833
Riboflavin	mg	0.602
Niacin	mg	3.472
Vitamin B-6	mg	0.232
Folate, DFE	µg	16
Vitamin B-12	µg	0
Vitamin A, RAE	µg	405
Vitamin A, IU	IU	8090
Vitamin D (D2 + D3)	µg	0
Vitamin D	IU	0
Fatty acids, total saturated	g	0.272
Fatty acids, total monounsaturated	g	0.285
Fatty acids, total polyunsaturated	g	0.213
Cholesterol	mg	0

Source: USDA Nutrient Database

Water Cress

Scientific name of watercress is *Nasturtium officinale*. Watercress belongs to the family *Brassicaceae*, the cabbage family (syn. Cruciferae). In other words, watercress is a brassica vegetable or a cruciferous vegetable.

Brassica vegetables are biennial in their growing habit but for food purposes they are grown as annuals. Brassica vegetables believed to be originated in the region comprising of Western Europe, the Mediterranean region and the temperate regions of Asia.

Watercress is a sun-loving, water-loving, trailing, perennial plant which grows well in an aquatic environment. Young tender leaves of watercress are used as a leafy vegetable. Leaves are serrated and with a mild spicy flavour. Leaves are cooked just like any other brassica vegetable such as kale leaves, seakale and broccoli leaves.

Like other brassica vegetables, watercress is rich in dietary fiber and antioxidant vitamins, Vitamin A and Vitamin C. Since it is rich in antioxidants, consumption of watercress is considered to be good to prevent the life style diseases such as cancer. It is also rich in minerals such as calcium, iodine, and iron.

Nutrition in Raw Watercress

Nutrient	Unit	Value per100g	1.0"cup, chopped"34.0g	1.0"sprig" 2.5g	10.0"sprigs"2 5.0g
Water	g	95.11	32.34	2.38	23.78
Energy	kcal	11	4	0	3
Protein	g	2.3	0.78	0.06	0.58
Total lipid (fat)	g	0.1	0.03	0	0.02
Carbohydrate, by difference	g	1.29	0.44	0.03	0.32
Fiber, total dietary	g	0.5	0.2	0	0.1
Sugars, total	g	0.2	0.07	0	0.05
Calcium, Ca	mg	120	41	3	30
Iron, Fe	mg	0.2	0.07	0	0.05
Magnesium, Mg	mg	21	7	1	5
Phosphorus, P	mg	60	20	2	15
Potassium, K	mg	330	112	8	82
Sodium, Na	mg	41	14	1	10
Zinc, Zn	mg	0.11	0.04	0	0.03
Vitamin C, total ascorbic acid	mg	43	14.6	1.1	10.8
Thiamin	mg	0.09	0.031	0.002	0.022
Riboflavin	mg	0.12	0.041	0.003	0.03
Niacin	mg	0.2	0.068	0.005	0.05
Vitamin B-6	mg	0.129	0.044	0.003	0.032
Folate, DFE	Åµg	9	3	0	2
Vitamin A, RAE	Åµg	160	54	4	40
Vitamin A, IU	IU	3191	1085	80	798
Vitamin E (alpha-tocopherol)	mg	1	0.34	0.02	0.25
Vitamin K (phylloquinone)	Åµg	250	85	6.2	62.5
Fatty acids, total saturated	g	0.027	0.009	0.001	0.007
Fatty acids, total monounsaturated	g	0.008	0.003	0	0.002
Fatty acids, total polyunsaturated	g	0.035	0.012	0.001	0.009

Source: USDA Nutrient Database

BIBLIOGRAPHY

Choudhary, B. (1992). *Vegetables*. New Delhi: National Book Trust of India

Nirmal K. Sinha, Ph.D, Y. H. Hui, E. Özgül Evranuz, Muhammad Siddiq, Jasim Ahmed (2011)*Handbook of Vegetables and Vegetable Processing* :Blackwell Publishing Ltd

Germplasm Resources Information Network . (2014, October Monday). Retrieved October Monday, 2014, from GRIN NPGS: http://www.ars-grin.gov/npgs/

Handbook of Agriculture. (2005). New Delhi: ICAR.

UC Davis Post Harvest. (2014, October Monday). Retrieved October Monday, 2014, from UC Davis Post Harvest Technology Center: http://postharvest.ucdavis.edu/producefacts/

USDA ARS . (2014, October Monday). Retrieved October Monday, 2014, from USDA Agricultural Research Service: http://www.ars.usda.gov/main/main.htm

USDA Nutrient Database . (2014, October Monday). Retrieved October Monday, 2014, from USDA Nutrient Database: http://ndb.nal.usda.gov/ndb/search/list

USDA Plant Database . (2014, October Monday). Retrieved October Monday, 2014, from USDA Plant Database: http://plants.usda.

www.ingramcontent.com/pod-product-compliance
Lightning Source LLC
Chambersburg PA
CBHW070359290526
45790CB00004B/1563